Living with Lupus

Unexplained pain and inflammation, general weakness, and sensitivity to light are just a few of the symptoms of one of the most baffling and chronic autoimmune diseases—lupus. Dr. Mark Horowitz, a noted rheumatologist, has written a complete guide to the whats, whys, and hows of this difficult illness that affects more than a half-million Americans. His compassionate, up-to-the-minute advice includes information on diagnoses, medications, and treatments, resource listings of books and organizations, and breakthrough medical and lifestyle options that bring not only hope but real help—enabling lupus sufferers to cope both physically and emotionally.

Mark Horowitz, M.D., is a rheumatologist with a private practice in New York City. He received his M.D. from Northeastern Ohio Universities College of Medicine and did his residency at the Mount Sinai Medical Center in New York City, where he was also a clinical instructor in the Department of Medicine. Marietta Abrams Brill is a freelance writer.

LIVING

WITH

Lupus

A Comprehensive Guide to
Understanding and Controlling Lupus
While Getting On with Your Life

MARK HOROWITZ, M.D.,
AND
MARIETTA ABRAMS BRILL

Illustrations by Kent Humphreys

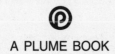

A PLUME BOOK

For Ronnie, whose words are with me always.
MAB

A NOTE TO THE READER
The ideas, procedures, and suggestions contained in this book are not intended as a substitute for consulting with your physician. All matters regarding your health require medical supervision.

PLUME
Published by the Penguin Group
Penguin Books USA Inc., 375 Hudson Street,
New York, New York 10014, U.S.A.
Penguin Books Ltd, 27 Wrights Lane, London W8 5TZ, England
Penguin Books Australia Ltd, Ringwood, Victoria, Australia
Penguin Books Canada Ltd, 10 Alcorn Avenue,
Toronto, Ontario, Canada M4V 3B2
Penguin Books (N.Z.) Ltd, 182–190 Wairau Road, Auckland 10, New Zealand

Penguin Books Ltd, Registered Offices:
Harmondsworth, Middlesex, England

First published by Plume, an imprint of Dutton Signet,
a division of Penguin Books USA Inc.

First Printing, April, 1994
10 9 8 7 6 5 4 3 2

 REGISTERED TRADEMARK—MARCA REGISTRADA

LIBRARY OF CONGRESS CATALOGING IN PUBLICATION DATA:
Horowitz, Mark.
  Living with lupus : a comprehensive guide to understanding and controlling lupus
while getting on with your life / Mark Horowitz and Marietta Abrams Brill : illustrations by Kent Humphreys.
     p. cm.
  ISBN 0-452-27056-1
  1. Systemic lupus erythematosus—Popular works.   I. Abrams Brill, Marietta.   II.
Title.
RC924.5.L85H67 1994
362.1'9677—dc20   93—21066
                                                                              CIP

Printed in the United States of America
Set in Century Expanded
Designed by Eve L. Kirch

Contents

PART I

Understanding Lupus

Making a New Start

Whether you've just learned that you have lupus, or you've been living with it for a while, you probably have many questions. You're not alone. Lupus erythematosus, commonly known simply as lupus, is harder to pin down than it is to pronounce. One day you may feel fine; the next you're struggling with a flare that puts you out of commission. Your symptoms may start out in one part of your body, only to shift to another. Lupus can affect many body systems, so your experience with lupus may be totally different from someone else's. And keeping an emotional balance—no easy task for even the healthiest of mortals—can be especially tricky when your physical well-being is so unstable.

It's not uncommon for people with lupus to go for months or years—from doctor to doctor, from test to test—before hearing the words "lupus erythematosus." Once it's finally given, the diagnosis of lupus unleashes mixed emotions. You may feel relieved at finally having a medical explanation for the confusing bundle of symptoms you've been experiencing. (They were *not* all in your head!) At the same time, a diagnosis may bring on a host of fears and anxieties about the unknown course your life will take.

Take heart. Lupus treatment has taken huge leaps forward over the past few decades. In the early 1950s, lupus was often fatal. Today, thanks to a deeper understanding of the disease, the majority of people with lupus can expect to live out a normal life-span. And many people can expect those years to be quite healthy and productive ones—if certain steps are taken.

Helping you make the most of your life with lupus is the goal of this book. Though lupus cannot be cured, it can be controlled. It's up to you, with the help of your doctor, to *take* control. And that starts with getting the most up-to-date information. Let's take a closer look at what you're dealing with.

Systemic Lupus Erythematosus Defined

Lupus is currently thought to be **a chronic systemic autoimmune disease that causes inflammation of various parts of the body.** What exactly does that mean?

A Chronic Disorder

"Chronic" means that the problem is long-term. Until there's a cure for lupus, you'll always be susceptible to its symptoms. Luckily, the symptoms usually are not constant, or they need not be with treatment. They **flare** and **remit**—come and go. For many people, with proper care, the periods of flare can be kept at bay for months or years at a time.

The idea of having a chronic disease probably sounds overwhelming, and it can be a challenge that requires great commitment and strength of spirit. But let's look at it in perspective. Back before effective treatment was available, lupus was thought to be an acute illness. And an acute attack of lupus symptoms was often fatal. Today, however, people are *living with* chronic lupus, not dying from acute attacks.

Systemic Effects

"Systemic" means that lupus can touch almost any body system, from the head to the muscles in the toes. Thankfully, no single person will have lupus in all parts of her or his body. Usually the disease targets only one or a few parts. In fact, for most people, the symptoms are mostly mild, rarely life-threatening. On the other hand, lupus of the kidney (or nephritis) and lupus of the nervous system can be very serious if left unchecked.

An Autoimmune Disease

Current thinking has it that lupus is an autoimmune disease—one that causes the body's immune system to fight itself, as well as outside invaders. In a way, the lupus immune system is overprotective. Antibodies are soldiers in the immune system's defense army. They normally target and trap harmful forces, such as bacteria and viruses. People with lupus can still defend against these threats. But for reasons unknown, their immune system also targets healthy parts of the body. This is called an autoimmune response: defending ("immune") against the self ("auto"). The misinformed immune sys-

tem then produces antibodies to the self, called autoantibodies, which triggers a chain reaction of defense tactics.
Inflammation is part of this disease.

Inflammation and Lupus

"Inflammation" comes from a Latin verb meaning to
kindle or set on fire. An inflamed body part takes on
some pretty fiery traits. It will often become red and hot,
may swell and may produce liquids. When "itis" is tagged
on to the end of a word, it's a code for inflammation. For
example, rhinitis means inflammation of the nasal passages; laryngitis means inflammation of the larynx. Inflammation is one of many processes the immune system
uses to protect the body from threatening forces. If you
get a sliver in your finger, you'll notice the area around
it getting red, swollen—inflamed. This is your body's way
of protecting itself from the foreign invader and ousting
it. A sore throat also looks red and feels swollen, a sign
that your body is fighting off bacteria.

An inflamed body part won't work as well as it does
under cooler conditions because the inflammation takes
priority over other functions. For example, when you
have a sore throat, it's more difficult to swallow; a swollen knee joint doesn't bend as easily as normal. And if inflammation continues in some parts of the body for long
periods, as can happen with lupus, permanent damage
can occur. That's why lupus treatment often aims to reduce inflammation.

Symptoms of Lupus

Symptoms vary from person to person. And they often build up slowly, starting with a mild, vague discomfort that turns into a specific symptom. When people are first diagnosed with lupus, they usually have symptoms such as fever, tiredness, appetite or weight loss, aches and pains, swollen glands, nausea, headache, depression, easy bruising, hair loss or swelling.

Also typical of lupus is a rash over the cheeks and bridge of the nose, in the shape of a butterfly. Other common skin symptoms include scaly, red, disc-shaped marks, painless ulcers in the mouth, bald spots, sun rashes and fingers that turn white or blue in the cold (also known as Raynaud's disease).

Your particular symptoms depend on the part or parts of the body affected by lupus. For example, if lupus strikes your skin, you may get a rash; if it afflicts your joints, you may feel a stiffness and heaviness in your limbs. In Chapter 3, "The Anatomy of Lupus," we'll examine which parts of the body are commonly affected by lupus, and how they are affected.

Different Types of Lupus

There is more than one type of lupus. Besides systemic lupus erythematosus (SLE), there is a type of lupus that only affects the skin, called discoid lupus (because it causes disc-shaped rashes), and a type that is caused by certain medicines, called drug-induced lupus. There are also rarer types of lupus that only affect infants or older people, and types that affect the skin in a different way from discoid lupus.

No Known Cause or Cure

The final word about lupus is not yet out. The cause is unknown, though several theories are now being researched. Experts think a few different paths may lead to the cause: hormones, genetics, viruses and even stress, together or separately, seem to play a role.

A cure for lupus still eludes us. Some researchers are even debating whether lupus is truly an autoimmune disease. But in a year (or two, or ten) our understanding of the disease may change for the better. A cause may be discovered, completely changing the definition of lupus and possibly bringing us closer to a cure. In the meantime, scientific experience with many patients tells us that certain steps can be taken to make lupus easier to live with.

What This Book Will Tell You

Living with Lupus presents the current knowledge about lupus so that you can make the best use of it. It has been written for those of you who are ready to take the next step in managing your disease. You'll learn the latest medical information to help you become an expert in lupus and options for its treatment. As advances are made in lupus, you'll be ready to understand what they mean.

You'll learn that the type of lupus you have will determine your treatment. All patients are unique in the way they react to lupus and the type of treatment that's right for them.

We'll look at lupus from the inside out. So that you can better understand the disease, we'll delve deeper into the process of immunity, how it seems to be led astray by lupus and how the disorder can affect different parts of the body. We'll help you separate the myths about lupus from the facts, and explore some of the reasons why it's so hard to diagnose.

Any chronic illness carries an emotional burden. Fear, anger and depression are just a few of the feelings suffered by people with an illness like lupus. These emotions are natural. They should not be ignored or pushed aside, but should be first accepted, then understood and dealt with. In Chapter 4 you'll find methods of coping with some of your feelings and the ways they affect your relationships, your career and other aspects of your life.

But getting a clear picture of lupus and its challenges is just half the story. The big question is, what can you *do* about it? The answer is, lots. In the second part of *Living with Lupus*, we'll give you a blueprint for action. We'll review the treatments most commonly used today, explaining how they work and what can be done to lessen their side effects. You'll also discover some proven hints for coping with the emotional and physical ups and downs of lupus, including practical ways of detecting and preventing flares.

One of the subjects that patients with lupus most frequently ask me about is pregnancy—and for good reason. Lupus strikes women nine times more often than men, and symptoms tend to peak during childbearing years. With a few exceptions, lupus should have little effect on your ability to have a healthy child. In Chapter 7, we'll examine what can be done to help ensure a healthy delivery for both mother and child. We'll even tackle some of the challenges of parenthood, which can be greater for women coping with lupus.

Finally, we'll look briefly into the future. What is the direction of new treatments? What paths are investigators following in search of a cause and a cure? These and other questions will be addressed in the last chapter.

CHAPTER 1

Lupus Lore vs. Reality

Right from the start, people have been misled by lupus. An early sign of this deception is seen in the name: lupus means "wolf" in Latin. It was first coined by a doctor in the 1200s to describe the skin marks sometimes seen in people with lupus. These lesions were similar to and might have been mistaken for the bite of a wolf.

Though misleading in one way—lupus has nothing to do with a wolf bite—the name is oddly appropriate. Like the fairy-tale wolf we all knew and loathed in "Little Red Riding Hood," lupus is a master of disguise. Nicknamed "the great imitator," lupus takes on the traits of many other diseases, depending on which part of the body it strikes. Lupus of the joints is often mistaken for arthritis; lupus of the lung can seem like a lung infection, and so on.

How, then, was lupus finally exposed for the systemic autoimmune disease it is known as today? The process was a slow one, and the search for the true identity of lupus continues today.

The Early Years

The first lupus experts never suspected a link between the "wolf bite" lesions on the skin and the internal symptoms of lupus. Lupus was known only as a type of erythematosus, or redness of the skin. It wasn't until 1872 that the Hungarian dermatologist Moritz Kaposi saw that lupus went more than skin deep. In 1895 the word "systemic" was added to "lupus erythematosus" by the Canadian physician Sir William Osler to describe the growing list of organs lupus afflicted.

Over the next fifty or so years, lupus was thought, wrongly, to be a type of cancer and, also wrongly, to be a type of tuberculosis. But experts continued adding to their list of organs and body parts targeted by lupus: the blood system, lungs, heart, joints, muscles, kidneys, brain and veins. (Fortunately, it's extremely rare for any one person to have lupus in all of these parts at once.)

The Modern Era: Tests and Treatments

A landmark in the history of lupus came in 1948 with the discovery of the lupus erythematosus (LE) cell. This was the first time problems with the immune system were suspected as a cause of lupus symptoms. The LE cell is found in the blood of some people with lupus. Its presence indicates an autoantibody. Antibodies are proteins in the blood that normally help fight off foreign, potentially dangerous cells; an autoantibody is an antibody that fights against cells of the self. When the LE cell was discovered, it was thought that only people with lupus had it. We now know that people with other autoimmune diseases, such as rheumatoid arthritis, also have the LE cell. Some people with lupus don't have the cell at all. The LE cell test has since been replaced by others for lupus.

On the heels of the LE cell test came more tests to help describe lupus and identify people who had it. One test, still used today, is a false-positive test for syphilis, also known as the phospholipid test. What does this mean? Some people with lupus who take the syphilis blood test show a positive result even though they don't have the disease. For some reason, about 30 percent of people with lupus will have a false-positive response to the syphilis test.

Another important test is actually a group of tests known as antinuclear antibody (ANA) tests. The ANA tests tell whether specific autoantibodies in the blood are fighting against healthy cells.

Many other tests have been developed in recent years. Some are used to help diagnose people with lupus. Others are used to keep track of their progress. But there's no single blood or urine test that says, "You do/do not have lupus." If your doctor suspects that you have a strep throat, the strep test will tell whether you do or don't. Testing for lupus is not that simple (not much about lupus is). We'll discuss the tests for lupus, and what they tell and don't tell, in Chapter 2, "Unmasking Lupus: Diagnosis."

With the discovery of corticosteroids in the mid-1950s, the treatment of systemic lupus took a quantum leap forward. Corticosteroids are the main treatment today for all types of systemic lupus. For skin reactions, antimalarial drugs are the mainstay. Therapies such as immunosuppressive drugs (drugs that calm down the immune system) are used for the more serious complications caused by lupus, including lupus nephritis.

The 1950s also uncovered a dark side of drugs and lupus. During this time a disease that closely resembled lupus became linked with hydralazine, a drug used to treat high blood pressure. This syndrome is now known as drug-induced lupus, or lupus caused by certain medicines.

Though medical experts today are getting a better handle on the nature and behavior of lupus, the wolf's disguises still fool many doctors. Even the most compassionate and knowledgeable of physicians can be led astray by the confusing symptoms.

And lupus is still completely baffling to most non-doctors. If they don't have lupus, or don't know someone who has it, most people would be hard-pressed to describe it. Or, even worse, they've "heard something about it—isn't it fatal?" That's just ignorance. The majority of people with lupus *can take control.*

Setting the Record Straight

It's up to us, the ones who have lupus or who care about people with lupus, to set the record straight. So, for the record ...

Some Lupus Statistics

Though most people you know have probably never heard of lupus, it's not all that uncommon. You may be surprised to discover that lupus strikes one out of every 2,000 Americans. About 500,000 Americans have been diagnosed with lupus; more than 16,000 new cases are reported every year. Lupus is more common than leukemia.

It's also more prevalent than muscular dystrophy or cerebral palsy, multiple sclerosis or cystic fibrosis.

Keep in mind that statistics are only as good as our methods for detecting the disease. The better we get at diagnosing lupus, the more people we'll uncover who have it. The fact that people are living longer with lupus also changes these statistics over time. Just fifty years ago, people may have died before they were ever diagnosed. Today, with earlier diagnosis and longer survival, there appear to be more of us with lupus.

The Lupus Bias

Lupus tends to discriminate. Women are nine times more likely to get lupus; about one in 700 American females have lupus. Lupus is three times more common among black women than white women. One out of every 245 black women have lupus. Black women also tend to have symptoms about six years earlier than white women. Lupus is also more prevalent among Asians, Hispanics and certain Native American groups. And, much to the dismay of many women, lupus tends to strike during the childbearing years (ages fourteen to forty-five). This has led experts to believe that female hormones play a role in causing lupus. Men, children and the elderly are not magically protected from lupus: they are affected, but less often.

Six Types of Lupus

You may be a little confused by the different ways we use the word "lupus." Sometimes it sounds like a skin disease. Sometimes it sounds like a systemic disease of different body parts. At still other times it sounds like a disease caused by drugs.

All of the above are true. "Lupus" is a general term that embraces six different disorders. Doctors have divided the general population of those with lupus into several groups based on how they get the disease, when they get it, the nature of their symptoms and how they're treated. All the people in these groups are said to have lupus because all of them have a similar problem with the immune system.

The six different types of lupus are systemic lupus erythematosus, discoid lupus, drug-induced lupus, neonatal syndrome, subacute cutaneous lupus erythematosus and late-onset lupus. Most people have either systemic lupus or discoid lupus.

1. Systemic lupus erythematosus (SLE) is a chronic inflammation of one or more different organs or body systems. Usually the disease starts out mildly, with vague symptoms. Tiredness, fever and weight loss are the usual early complaints. It's easy at first to shrug them off as a common problem, such as flu or stress. And many doctors will take a "wait and see" approach. Sure enough, the problem often passes—only to return. The come-and-go pattern of lupus is one of its trademarks: the disease occurs in cycles of flare (activity) and remission (rest).

Lupus can strike almost any part of the body. We'll take a closer look at the ways it can strike in Chapter 3. Most of the symptoms are shared by other diseases, but some, such as the butterfly or malar rash ("malar" means pertaining to the cheek or side of the head), are seen almost exclusively in people with systemic lupus.

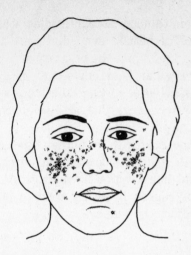

The malar, or butterfly rash, common in systemic lupus, covers the cheeks and nose.

2. Discoid lupus (lupus of the skin) is limited to the skin. Discoid lupus was named for the disc-shaped rashes, usually no more than two inches across, raised and scaly, that spread across the nose and cheeks and sometimes the chest or scalp. Sometimes discoid lupus is only a reddish rash, which can make diagnosis confusing because such a rash could be caused by a number of different conditions. Performing a skin biopsy—examining a sample of the skin under a microscope—is the only way of making an accurate diagnosis.

3. Drug-induced lupus is an adverse reaction to some prescription drugs that produces symptoms of lupus. An estimated 15,000 to 20,000 cases are reported each year in the United States. Luckily, lupus of this sort is reversible: the symptoms gradually disappear after the patient stops taking the medication.

For reasons not yet known, certain drugs trigger the

immune system to make autoantibodies, which results in
inflammation. The best-known culprits are hydralazine, a
drug used to treat high blood pressure, and procainamide, for irregular heartbeats, but as many as fifty
drugs are suspected of setting off a lupus syndrome. Table 1 outlines the drugs that are well-documented pro-
vokers of lupus.

As is *not* the case with any other type of lupus, men,
children and the elderly share the same risk as women of
getting a lupus-like reaction from drugs. Also, the symptoms of lupus caused by drugs tend to be milder, and
they rarely affect the kidneys.

Table 1. Drugs that Can Cause Lupus

Strong Association Between Drug and Lupus

Drug	Main Use
Chlorpromazine	Psychiatric disturbances
Hydralazine	High blood pressure
Isoniazid	Tuberculosis
Methyldopa	High blood pressure
Procainamide	Irregular heartbeat

Possible Association Between Drug and Lupus

Drug	Main Use
Acebutolol	High blood pressure
Atenolol	High blood pressure
Captopril	High blood pressure
Carbamazepine	Seizure disorders
Ethosuximide	Seizure disorders
Labetalol	High blood pressure
Levadopa	Parkinson's disease
Lithium carbonate	Mental disturbances
Mephenytoin	Convulsions
Metoprolol	High blood pressure

Nitrofurantoin	Infection
Oxyprenolol	High blood pressure
Penicillamine	Rheumatoid arthritis/scleroderma
Phenytoin	Seizure disorders
Primidone	Seizure disorders
Quinidine	Irregular heartbeat
Trimethadion	Convulsions

4. Neonatal lupus is a rare type of lupus that affects newborn infants—but experts think the occurrence of the problem is underestimated. It can take the form of a skin rash, changes in the blood or heart block.

Skin symptoms begin as a scaly, red, bumpy rash, which breaks out after the child goes out in the sun. These lesions usually disappear within six or twelve months, with little evidence that they ever existed.

Blood problems (in medicalese, dyscrasias) include anemia, low white blood cell count and low platelet count. Until they disappear (usually within a few months) these symptoms are often so mild that they don't need to be treated.

Heart block is the most serious problem of neonatal lupus. This is a condition in which the electrical impulses that trigger a heartbeat are slowed or blocked, causing the heart rate to become very low, which can be extremely serious. But most babies can be treated and will grow normally.

If you're a woman with lupus, your risk of having a baby with neonatal heart block is about one in twenty. If you also have a specific kind of autoantibody called anti-Ro antibody (so named because the autoantibody was first found in a person whose name began with "Ro"), the risk increases. Women with lupus who want to get pregnant definitely should be screened for the anti-Ro antibody.

5. Subacute cutaneous lupus erythematosus (SCLE) is a milder form of both discoid and systemic lupus. The skin lesions may start out as small red discs or pimples which expand and merge, just like discoid lesions. But they don't leave scars. The sun is a major cause of SCLE skin symptoms, so sun exposure should be limited.

The systemic symptoms of SCLE usually include muscle and joint pain, fever and general discomfort. Serious kidney or nervous system problems are rare.

6. Late-onset lupus is a type of lupus seen in people over the age of fifty. It's estimated that up to 20 percent of people with lupus have late-onset lupus. Late-onset lupus is mostly a female disease, but it's less discriminating than systemic or discoid disease: about one-third of those who suffer from late-onset lupus are men. People who get lupus in their fifth decade or later have the same range of symptoms as those with SLE, but they're milder. As with neonatal lupus, serious kidney and central nervous system problems are quite rare.

Questions and Answers About Lupus

Before we go any further in your lupus lesson—and get into the nitty-gritty of what causes the disease—let's answer some common questions.

Q. Is lupus contagious?

A. No. There is no reason to quarantine yourself from other people, or to keep away from people with lupus. If lupus were contagious, the close friends and physicians of people with lupus would also get the disease. This simply doesn't happen.

In trying to uncover a cause for lupus, researchers have collected some evidence that viruses may play a role. But the concept of a lupus virus is still just that—a concept. Investigators have yet to pinpoint a specific viral organism. And even if lupus is caused by a virus, that doesn't mean the virus is contagious. As it stands, you can't catch lupus in the way that, say, you can catch a cold. Experts think a combination of factors may be at work in causing lupus. Certain people may be at higher risk of getting lupus because of their genetic makeup. This leads us to the next question.

Q. Is lupus inherited?

A. People do not inherit lupus in the same way they inherit hemophilia or sickle-cell anemia or Tay-Sachs disease. With these diseases, there is a strong genetic link between parent and child. With lupus, only 5 percent of families show a true family connection—that is, the disease develops in the child of a person with the disease.

This statistic doesn't rule out a genetic role. We know that the way an individual's immune system responds can be inherited. Some relatives of people with lupus show signs of similar immune system problems. As a group, they're more likely to have rheumatoid arthritis than relatives of people without lupus. Like lupus, rheumatoid arthritis is an immune disorder that causes inflammation of the joints.

Also, autoantibodies are detected in healthy family members of people with lupus. Autoantibodies are evident in almost all people with lupus (as well as many people who do not have lupus). Some doctors think these healthy family members also have a gene that protects them from lupus.

These and other findings lead experts to believe that people may inherit a *susceptibility* to lupus—and that environmental factors take over from there. You may be genetically prone to getting lupus, but that alone won't be enough for you to become ill. It may take something like exposure to sunlight or a certain drug or, as discussed above, a virus to trigger an immune response and flare.

Q. Is lupus fatal?
A. Discoid lupus is not fatal. And even though lupus cannot be cured, the vast majority of people with systemic lupus can control their symptoms so that they're not life-threatening. Today 90 percent survive lupus, and the life-span seems to approach that of the average population. The reasons: people seek treatment earlier; therapy has become more effective; and there are more caregivers familiar with lupus and its treatment than ever before.

Although it's uncommon, some people do die from lupus. Of these, most have severe disease—usually involving the kidneys or a system-wide infection. Usually the serious infection does not result from the disease, but is a complication related to immunosuppressive therapy.

On the other end of the spectrum, up to 20 percent of people with systemic lupus go for months or years without any symptoms or any need for treatment. There doesn't seem to be a reason for these remissions, or disease-free periods. People have been known to be in remission for twenty years or longer. Remissions seem to be more likely after flares involving the skin or joints.

They're less common after the kidneys, lungs, heart, gastrointestinal tract or nervous system have been involved.

Q. Can I have children?

A. Most women with lupus can have successful pregnancies. While discoid lupus carries few risks to the mother or child, systemic lupus pregnancies are considered high-risk. This may sound frightening, but treating a pregnancy as though it were a high-risk one is mainly a preventive measure. In about 50 percent of lupus pregnancies, the mother's health is not affected by pregnancy, and the pregnancy is not endangered by lupus. But because problems can't always be predicted, it's best to play it safe and consult closely with a doctor skilled in caring for women with problematic pregnancies.

Some of the problems women with lupus may face during pregnancy include toxemia, a high miscarriage rate and premature deliveries. We'll discuss these in more detail in Chapter 7.

As a general rule, women with severe high blood pressure or serious kidney problems should avoid pregnancy altogether because the risks to the mother are considered too great. *But each woman is different.* If you want to become pregnant—even if you have kidney or blood pressure problems—it's best to talk with your doctor.

Q. Why is lupus more common in women than in men?

A. We don't have a final answer to this question. Some studies suggest that estrogen may make women more susceptible to problems related to the immune system. Estrogen, the female hormone made by the ovaries, plays a key role in a woman's ability to have children. This theory may help explain why lupus is more prevalent in women of childbearing age.

Q. Are humans the only mammals that have lupus?
A. Several animals develop illnesses that resemble lupus. A type of mouse called the New Zealand black mouse sometimes shows autoantibodies, anemia and kidney inflammation. Young adult dogs have exhibited symptoms of lupus, including the butterfly rash. (In fact, former President Bush's dog, Millie, suffers from lupus.) Elephants are known to have lupus. And a certain strain of mink, known by its dark blue coat, has a lupus-like syndrome. Wolves don't seem to show the symptoms of their namesake disease.

Q. Will I ever lead a normal life?
A. To lead a "normal life," your challenge is to become as comfortable as possible with this lifetime companion. Accept lupus as a part of your life, and accept your role as your body's primary caretaker. You will have flares. And you probably will have periods of remission.

It's up to you (with the help of your doctor) to tune in to your body and learn what kindles your flares. It's up to you to take steps that will help you dodge these triggering events. If you learn that sunlight ignites a flare, you don't have to cower indoors; you can wear sunscreens and protective clothing. Take care of your body and it will repay you with fewer flares.

No one says this will be easy. But you *can* strike a truce with lupus. You don't have to do it alone—and you shouldn't. Your doctor is there to help you manage your disease in whatever way he or she can. Family members and friends may feel better knowing what you need and how they can support you. Lupus groups have formed across the country to educate and support you. (See "Resources" at the end of this book.) All you have to do is ask.

Every person with lupus has her or his own way of

coping with the disease. What's normal for you may not
be comfortable for someone else. You must find your own
balance. We hope the chapters that follow will help show
you how.

CHAPTER 2

Unmasking Lupus: Diagnosis

Eight years is a long time to live with pain and uncertainty. But that's been cited as the *average* time it takes to reach a diagnosis of systemic lupus. And as you may know, the road to diagnosis is not only slow, but can also be rough. Along the way, lupus sufferers are likely to travel some foreign and unfriendly territory: emergency rooms, testing clinics and the offices of confused or skeptical physicians and even psychiatrists. You've probably endured more prodding, pinpricking and picture-taking than you did in the entire pre-lupus era of your life. Consider yourself lucky if you had a physician to take charge and help guide you through the referrals and the flurry of tests. Many people go it alone.

Unfortunately, the results of these visits often prove a diagnostic dead end. Depending on the symptoms, false diagnoses range from arthritis to muscular dystrophy to cancer to one of the most dreaded of all: hypochondria. There's little worse than suffering—sometimes to the point of immobility—and not being taken seriously. Not knowing what's wrong is painful; not being believed can be a form of torture.

It's no wonder people greet a diagnosis as serious as lupus with some relief—relief at knowing that there *are* doctors who understand, at the prospect of eased pain, at being believed. But this relief does not come without some casualties, one being the bank account. The multitude of tests and visits to physicians can take a huge toll on anyone's savings.

And the relief of diagnosis isn't enough to erase feelings of mistrust, anger and self-doubt: "Don't doctors know the symptoms of lupus?" "Even my family thought I was inventing symptoms!" "Why wasn't I more assertive? I brought this on myself!" "Why must diagnosis be so difficult?"

It's natural to want to cast blame—on the medical profession, on yourself, on your loved ones. (We'll address this issue in Chapter 4, "Emotional Trials and Triumphs.") Though some of this blame may be warranted, the biggest culprit is often the disease itself. There's good reason lupus is called "the great imitator," "the impostor disease" and "the disease with a thousand faces." Lupus is a tricky disease—trickier than most—to diagnose.

How Diseases Are Diagnosed: Start with a Theory

To diagnose any disease, doctors turn into detectives. Based on their patients' symptoms and their own experience, doctors start out with a theory about what's at the root of the problem. Like most good detectives, they

gather clues—from medical tests, trial therapies, observation—until they can prove that theory.

Rather than settle for a half-proven diagnosis, most
doctors will keep testing and watching until the clinical
picture sharpens to the point where there's little doubt
about the cause. Their conservative attitude is based on
the idea that a wrong diagnosis can have far worse effects than no diagnosis: it leads to unnecessary (and potentially dangerous) treatment and allows the real
disease to progress unchecked.

With most illnesses, the symptoms fall into neat, well-
defined categories, and the diagnostic process is relatively short and direct. Lupus throws a few kinks into
the diagnostic works.

What Makes Lupus So Hard to Diagnose?

As we mentioned, **the early symptoms of lupus are
not very specific.** These nonspecific symptoms, as doctors call them, are seen in lots of other illnesses. Classi-
fied as constitutional symptoms because they affect the
whole body, they include swollen glands, fatigue, fever
and weight loss. Lupus is probably not the first illness
that comes to most doctors' minds when a patient arrives
with these symptoms.

Even symptoms specific to lupus can lead doctors
astray. Swelling in the joints will make most doctors
think of arthritis before lupus; painful breathing may
raise suspicions of a lung infection, and so on. Doctors
must rule out the more common conditions before sus-
pecting other causes.

**The intensity of the symptoms seems to increase
gradually.** At first, you may feel only mild, vague symp-

toms, which seem to disappear. New symptoms then take hold, layering over the old ones. It can take months or years before your symptoms settle into a pattern or become bad enough for you to take notice. Convincing a doctor that your vague, shifting symptoms are not just everyday aches and pains can be a frustrating challenge.

Also, **lupus symptoms are elusive.** They typically follow a come-and-go pattern of flares and remissions, making them difficult to describe or show to your doctor.

Consider this example of a typical patient: Ellen had been feeling tired, but shrugged it off as overwork. Then one day she got a rash on her skin. At first she thought it would just go away (she didn't even suspect it was related to how tired she'd been feeling). She waited a few weeks before calling her doctor. Then she had to wait a few days more for the appointment. By the time her appointment date arrived, the rash was gone. Her doctor had to rely on a description of the rash rather than a firsthand view.

The same type of problem attends pain. Ellen's description of a pain she has right now will be more accurate than her description of a pain she had two weeks ago.

There is no typical lupus patient. Systemic lupus travels under a number of disguises: it can affect almost any part of the body, in a variety of combinations. And chances are your symptoms will differ from another's. This makes it difficult for doctors to recognize lupus readily.

Finally, **there is no single lupus test.** Just as there is no single symptom that points to lupus, no single blood or urine test says whether a person does or doesn't have lupus. Although tests do exist to *aid* in diagnosing lupus (see "Tests, Tests and More Tests" later in this chapter), they must be interpreted in light of your symptoms and your doctor's observations. Tests are just one part of the diagnostic puzzle.

As you can see, this mysterious disease can lead doctors into a diagnostic maze. How, then, is a diagnosis ever reached?

The Eleven Criteria for Lupus Diagnosis

Experts have pondered for many years about the best way formally to diagnose lupus. The National Lupus Foundation recommends that doctors take a broad view of each patient, which involves three steps: evaluate the symptoms, evaluate the immune system and then evaluate the two together.

To help doctors do this, the American College of Rheumatology has developed a list of eleven abnormalities that should raise a red flag for lupus. **At some point in their disease history, individuals must have had at least four—any four—of these eleven abnormalities to be diagnosed with lupus.** You don't have to have four of them at once. You could have had some symptoms months or even years ago, and could show evidence of others today. These conditions include physical symptoms that you feel and laboratory signs—or changes in laboratory tests—that reflect problems not readily felt by you or seen by your doctor.

1. Butterfly (malar) rash
2. Discoid lupus
3. Photosensitivity
4. Mucosal ulcers
5. Arthritis
6. Pleuritis/pericarditis

7. Nephritis
8. Central nervous system involvement
9. Blood disorders
10. Immunologic abnormalities
11. Antinuclear antibody

How do you know whether you meet these criteria? Let's take a closer look at what the American College of Rheumatology had in mind when it developed the list.

1. **A butterfly (malar) rash** is a red rash, either raised or flat, that covers the nose and cheeks. The distinctive pattern points very strongly to a diagnosis of lupus, since it's typical of so few other diseases.

2. **Discoid lupus,** described in detail in Chapter 1, is a scaly, red, disc-shaped raised rash that usually breaks out on the upper torso—face, neck, scalp, ears, chest and arms. Sunlight may trigger it.

3. **Photosensitivity** literally means sensitivity to light. It's a skin reaction that happens after exposure to ultraviolet (UV) light from the sun or even from fluorescent bulbs.

4. **Mucosal ulcers** are painless small sores on the inside of the mouth (usually the roof) or in the nostrils. Because they are painless, the ulcers may come and go unnoticed.

5. **Arthritis** is one of the few symptoms shared by almost all people with lupus. Pain and swelling in the joints of the arms, legs, hands, wrists, elbows or knees are typical, often shifting around from one joint to another (doctors refer to the pain as being migratory). The discomfort is also fleeting—it can come and go very quickly. The permanent crippling disfigurement feared with arthritis is not common with lupus.

6. **Pleuritis and pericarditis** are two related, but different, symptoms that often occur in people with lupus. Pleuritis means inflammation of the pleura, the lining of the lungs. Pericarditis is inflammation of the pericardium, or lining of the heart.

7. **Nephritis** means inflammation of the kidneys. The kidneys are the body's intricate filtration system; they help separate waste from nutrition and keep a healthy balance of fluids flowing through the body.

8. **Central nervous system involvement** means seizures or psychoses, frightening-sounding symptoms of systemic lupus—but they can be completely reversed with treatment. Seizures are the most common symptom. Psychoses, or mental disturbances, can take a variety of forms, from delusions to depression. Treatment depends on the cause. Since people may have neurologic problems that are not related to lupus, it's especially important to rule out other causes.

9. **Blood disorders** are caused by antibodies to different types of blood cells, resulting in abnormalily low concentrations of these cells in the blood. Changes may result in symptoms that you feel—or they may come and go without any outward evidence.

- **Anemia** is a lower level of red blood cells—the oxygen and nutrition-carrying cells of the body. The red blood cells either die prematurely or are manufactured too slowly within the bone marrow. Fatigue is the most common symptom.

- **Thrombocytopenia** is a lower amount of platelets, the cell particles responsible for clotting. Bleeding and easy bruising can result.

- **Leukopenia,** or a low white cell count, usually causes no adverse symptoms.

10. **Immunologic abnormalities** are detected by blood tests that measure autoantibodies, or antibodies to the self. Today there are four different tests for autoantibodies included in the immunologic group of tests, or workup. A person must test positive for only one of them to fulfill the immunologic requirement. These four tests, listed below, are discussed in more depth in the next section of this chapter.

- **Lupus erythematosus (LE) cell preparation test,** or, as doctors call it, LE Prep. The LE cell was one of the first cells identified in the blood of people with lupus that implicated the immune system in the disease process. An LE Prep is positive if the cell exists in the blood. The test has been replaced by other tests.

OR

- **Anti-double-stranded DNA antibody (also known as anti-DNA or anti-dsDNA).** DNA is short for dioxyrubonucleic acid, the component of every living cell that tells it what to do and how to do it. People with lupus develop antibodies to both single-stranded DNA (ss-DNA) and double-stranded DNA (ds-DNA). Detection of these anti-DNA antibodies in higher than normal quantities meets the immunologic requirement. A high anti-DNA level could forewarn of a flare, or of nephritis.

OR

- **Anti-Sm antibody (anti-Smith)** was so-called because the autoantibody was first found in a woman named Smith. Having anti-Sm antibody is considered

very "diagnostic" because this antibody is found only
in people with lupus. But not all people with lupus
have the anti-Sm antibody.

OR

- **False-positive test for syphilis** means that a person tests positive for having syphilis even though
she or he never had the disease. An autoantibody to
phospholipids, materials that form the outer part of
cells, is what throws off the syphilis test and gener-
ates the false-positive result.

11. **Antinuclear antibody (ANA)**—Almost every person with systemic lupus has antibodies to the nuclei (the
innermost cores) of cells, but so do people with some
other conditions. This means that a negative ANA is a
good test to rule out lupus, but a positive result isn't a
reliable way of confirming lupus.

Some common lupus symptoms—for example, vascular
disease or muscle weakness—didn't make the list. That
doesn't mean they're not caused by lupus, or that they're
less important. The eleven criteria were put together to
help doctors make a diagnosis; they are by no means a
complete list of lupus symptoms. (That list could fill a medical textbook—and has.) We'll explore these and other
symptoms of lupus in more detail in the next chapter.
Some of the eleven criteria are more "diagnostic" than
others. In other words, on their own, certain signs may
weigh more strongly as evidence of lupus. For example,
joint pain is a symptom of many different diseases, but
it's a common one in lupus. A positive autoantibody test
result is also very diagnostic, but autoantibody tests
aren't done routinely (they're never performed unless
your doctor already suspects lupus or a similar disease).

Tests, Tests and More Tests

Since systemic lupus wears so many masks, doctors rely heavily on the objective results of laboratory tests and other diagnostic procedures (such as X rays) for a clearer picture of what's going on inside.

Tests are used to help diagnose lupus, to help measure its effects on the body and to help predict where it will strike. Even after you've been diagnosed, it's important to make sure that the symptoms are caused by lupus—not by another problem that calls for different care. Once it's been diagnosed, it's easy to blame lupus for so many different symptoms and overlook the real problem. When your symptoms are nonspecific (which means that the symptoms could have many different causes), your doctor may have you take tests to narrow down the possibilities. This process is called differential diagnosis.

Some of these tests are very common; laboratories across the world do routine blood tests such as a serum creatinine, urinalysis, complete blood count (CBC) and complement.

Other tests are more specialized, custom-made for people with lupus and related diseases, such as scleroderma and Sjogren's syndrome. The ANA and other autoantibody tests fall into this category. The methods for these special tests may not be well defined. The possibility for error, which exists with even the most routine tests, is higher with the autoantibody tests. For this reason, you may have to take the tests more than once.

All this testing can be very confusing and frustrating if you don't understand the reasons for it and what the results mean. We've included a form at the end of this chapter to help you keep track of your tests. Also, the price of tests can mount, adding unwanted pressure to your life. Feel free to ask your doctor about the costs before you take the tests. If you know in advance, you may be able to plan for the expense. It's one small way of taking more control over your illness.

Below we've outlined some of the tests and procedures often prescribed for people with lupus either to help diagnose or to monitor the disease.

Autoantibodies

Autoantibodies seem to be the crystal balls of lupus, guiding the way to diagnosis and treatment when symptoms lead doctors astray. Experts aren't sure why, but specific autoantibodies seem to precede specific symptoms, or warn of a flare. But like most methods of foretelling the future, they aren't always accurate. Even so, they're among the best clues doctors have to the mysterious workings of lupus.

Antinuclear antibody (ANA). Antinuclear antibodies (ANA) are antibodies to the nuclei (center) of cells in the body. Every cell has a nucleus, so the ANA test will pick up many different kinds of autoantibodies. ANA is found in most people who have lupus, but it's also detected in many people who don't. This includes people with other autoimmune diseases of connective tissues (rheumatic diseases), healthy relatives of people with lupus, and older people.

ANA is a blood test in which serum is placed on a slide and a fluorescent dye is added. If antibody is present, it will glow. If the ANA test is positive, the blood sample will be diluted in half and examined again. If antibody still glows, the sample will be diluted again (into eighths) and examined. This process continues until the ANA is so diluted that it can't be detected. This highest dilution is called the titer—the outer limit of detection. The weaker the dilution that glows (fluoresces), the higher the ANA titer. Usually it takes a relatively high ANA titer to confirm a lupus diagnosis. Lower titers may suggest other autoimmune diseases, such as rheumatoid arthritis.

Doctors also look closely at the pattern of fluorescence to help distinguish among different autoimmune disorders. For example, a ring pattern—with fluorescence around the edges of nuclei—is the strongest indicator of systemic lupus. This pattern is seen in people with active disease, especially those with nephritis.

Certain prescription drugs in the bloodstream may cause false-positive results of the ANA test. These include hydralazine (used for high blood pressure) and procainamide.

Anti-double-stranded DNA antibody (anti-DNA, anti-dsDNA). Antibodies to DNA are tightly linked with lupus; they're seen in 40 to 75 percent of people with lupus, and in few other disorders. The presence of ds-DNA (double-stranded DNA) seems to indicate lupus nephritis. Rising levels warn of a flare.

Antibodies to ss-DNA (single-stranded DNA) are even more common among lupus sufferers; 90 to 95 percent of people will have this autoantibody. But people with other diseases have it, too.

Anti-Sm antibody (anti-Smith) and anti-nRNP. Anti-Sm was named after the first person known to have it; anti-nRNP stands for antinuclear ribonucleoprotein, which causes the antibody reaction. About 25 to 30 percent of people with systemic lupus have anti-Sm. Though not a strong connection, anti-Sm may indicate a comparatively mild course of nephritis, if nephritis exists at all.

Anti-nRNP is seen in about 40 percent of people with lupus. Anti-nRNP is generally seen as a mixed sign: though it signals lupus, it may foretell of myocarditis or other connective tissue diseases, such as rheumatoid arthritis, scleroderma and Sjogren's syndrome.

Anti-Ro and anti-La antibody. These autoantibodies, named after the people first known to have them, are often found together. About 40 percent of people with lupus have anti-Ro; it often shows up in people with lupus who test negative for ANA.

Anti-Ro is also found in people with subacute cutaneous lupus erythematosus (SCLE). It's also seen in women who give birth to children with neonatal lupus, as well as those who lack one of the complement proteins in their blood. (See page 40 for an explanation of *complement*.)

Antiphospholipid (anticardiolipin) antibodies. About 30 percent of people with lupus have antibodies to a part of cell walls called phospholipid. We discussed earlier how these autoantibodies are detected by the syphilis test, causing false-positive results. Antiphospholipid is also called anticardiolipin and, wrongly, lupus anticoagulant. But antiphospholipid/anticardiolipin is not an anticoagulant at all. In fact, it seems to have an opposite effect: instead of causing bleeding, it's more likely to cause excessive clotting. This can lead to serious problems such as thrombophlebitis (clots in the veins), which can in turn lead to gangrene of the hands or feet, arterial thromboses (clots in the arteries), low platelet counts and a propensity for miscarriage. Stroke and some forms of anemia are other problems related to antiphospholipid antibody.

Table 2. What the Autoantibodies Mean

Autoantibody	% of People with Systemic Lupus Who Have It	Lupus Symptoms Possibly Indicated	Other Diseases with Autoantibodies
ANA	90–95	None in particular	Many rheumatic diseases (rheumatoid arthritis, Sjogren's syndrome, etc.)
Anti-dsDNA	40–60	Nephritis	Few
Anti-ssDNA	90–95	None in particular	Many
Anti-nRNP	40–50	Raynaud's disease, myositis	Many
Anti-Ro	25–40	Sensitivity to light	SCLE, Sjogren's syndrome, neonatal lupus, complement deficiency
Antiphospho-lipid (a.k.a. anticardiolipin)	Unknown	Thrombosis, miscarriage	

Adapted with permission from Carolyn Ziminski, M.D., and *The Maryland Medical Journal* 1991, 40 (10):901–8.

Biopsy

Biopsy means the detailed examination of a piece of tissue taken from the body. In lupus, biopsy is often used to help diagnose skin problems such as discoid lesions (requiring a skin biopsy) and kidney problems such as nephritis (requiring a renal biopsy).

The skin biopsy involves removing a small piece of skin. This is usually done in the doctor's office. The doctor might numb the area with a local anaesthetic and, using a small, extremely sharp scalpel, remove a small bit of skin. A scar could result.

A renal (kidney) biopsy, on the other hand, usually takes place in the hospital (on an outpatient basis) under local anaesthesia, possibly with sedation. The patient lies flat while the doctor injects a long needle into one or both kidneys to remove a sample of tissue. The entire procedure takes about fifteen minutes.

A muscle biopsy may be needed to determine whether an inflammatory process is under way in myositis (muscle soreness).

Complement

Complement is a series of twenty or more proteins in the blood that are part of the immune system. Complement 4 (C4) and Complement 3 (C3) are among the more important parts of the complement system.

If levels of complement in the blood are low, it may mean that the complement system is busy attacking antibody-antigen complexes, and causing inflammation. As a result, low levels often reflect active lupus.

Complete Blood Count (CBC)

A CBC is a routine laboratory test for different blood cells: white blood cell (WBC), hemoglobin (Hgb), hematocrit (Hct) and platelet count. White blood cells help fight off infection; low levels may mean infection. Also, for reasons not completely understood, people with lupus often have lower than normal white blood count levels even without infection.

Hgb is a part of red cells that carries oxygen to body tissues. Hct measures the amount of red blood cells. Chronic inflammation, as is seen with lupus, can result in abnormal levels of Hgb.

Along with a positive ANA, a low white blood cell count, hematocrit or platelet count are often found in lupus. Monitoring these cell counts helps doctors keep track of lupus after it has been diagnosed.

Computerized Tomography (CT Scan/ CAT Scan)

The CT scan is like a very powerful X ray, helping doctors look closely at cysts and tumors. Like an X ray, the CT scan uses radiation to scan an image of the body, but in much smaller quantities. The patient lies on a table while a scanner circles around. The CT scan focuses a beam of radiation to create pictures of cross sections of the body. The beams then feed into a computer, which translates them into an image on the computer screen. Various shades of black-to-white match up with tissue density: white is bone, black is air, gray is liquid. The scan takes about twenty minutes.

Creatinine

Creatinine is a natural waste product created by the breakdown of muscle tissues. It is normally cleared from the body by the kidneys. But when the kidneys aren't functioning well, creatinine may remain in the body in higher levels. In people with lupus, it's often used to help doctors tell the degree of kidney damage caused by inflammation.

Electrocardiogram (ECG)

Sharp pains while inhaling might mean pericarditis (inflammation of the pericardium, the lining of the heart), but your doctor will first want to make sure it's not caused by other cardiac problems, such as angina or even an impending heart attack.

The ECG will help. The procedure is painless: metal discs attached to wires are taped to your chest. These probes transcribe the heart's electrical impulses into spiked patterns on paper. Damaged heart tissue gives off unsteady electrical signals, showing up as an abnormal electrocardiogram. An ECG is also vital in monitoring irregular heartbeat.

Electroencephalogram (EEG/Brain Wave)

The electrical activity of the brain can tell doctors a lot about its health; the EEG records electrical impulses to help doctors distinguish among diseases such as epilepsy, tumors and some psychological disorders.

Electrodes are pasted to the scalp (hair does *not* need to be shaved), transmitting a weak electrical current and recording its effects on the brain. A faint tingling sensation is not uncommon. The procedure lasts about an hour.

Electromyelogram (EMG)

In much the same way as an ECG picks up heart damage from changes in electrical patterns, the EMG detects muscle damage. A specific electrical pattern can be detected in damaged muscle.

Enzymes

Chemical enzymes are measured from a blood sample to help determine muscle damage. Higher than normal levels are associated with myositis. The higher above normal they are, the greater the damage. These tests not only help in diagnosis, but aid in monitoring response to therapy.

Glucose 6-Phosphate Dehydrogenase (G6PD)

G6PD is an enzyme that's found in red blood cells and is measured from a sample of blood. A lack of this enzyme may predispose to hemolytic anemia, one of the blood problems encountered by people with lupus. Hemolytic anemia is also aggravated by antimalarial drugs, which are often prescribed for discoid lupus.

Magnetic Resonance Imaging (MRI)

This sophisticated technology is used to identify inflammation, tumors, strokes and infections. It's particularly helpful in diagnosing problems with the pericardium, the lining of the heart, which are otherwise difficult to pinpoint. The patient lies in a tunnel-shaped tube for about five minutes. During this time, a startling noise of grating metal can be heard. Using radio waves and magnetic fields, the MRI constructs a three-dimensional image of the part of the body being studied. A painless procedure, MRI is considered safer than X ray. People with metallic implants, such as pacemakers, cannot undergo MRI.

Urine Tests

A urine sample is analyzed to detect any abnormal substances that warn of nephritis. These substances include protein and high levels of white blood cells and/or red blood cells. A negative urinalysis (the absence of these abnormalities) pretty much rules out nephritis.

A twenty-four-hour urine test will give doctors a more in-depth look at how well the kidneys are functioning. This simply means that urine samples are collected throughout the day.

Nephritis is nearly symptom-free in its early stages. The only way to tell whether you are developing the problem is by laboratory tests. People with lupus often will have their urine analyzed regularly to pick up this potentially dangerous condition in its early stages.

Ultrasound

Doctors may use ultrasound to visualize the movement of soft tissues, such as the heart, inside the body. The area being studied is covered with a lubricant (if it's your heart, your chest will be lubricated). A microphone is passed over the area, sending out sound waves and picking up their echoes. A computer visualizes these sonic messages.

X Ray

A chest X ray is often used to diagnose pleuritis (inflammation of the lining of the lung) and to rule out other conditions. During an X ray, radiation is passed through the body, creating a picture of the lung. A lung X ray can help rule out infection or structural problems that may be causing pleuritis-like chest pain. X rays are also used to differentiate lupus symptoms from true arthritis symptoms and to help keep track of lupus arthritis.

Table 3. Uses of Common Laboratory Tests in Lupus

Name of Test	What Is Being Tested
Blood urea nitrogen (BUN)	Kidney function
Creatinine	Kidney function
Calcium/phosphorus	Kidney function
Bilirubin	Liver function
Aminotransferase enzymes	Injury to liver, muscles, heart, hepatitis, kidney disease
Uric acid	Kidney disease
Lipids	Coronary artery disease

Depending on your particular symptoms, your doctor may need to monitor other parts of your body using pro-

cedures not mentioned here. Keep in mind that these
tests are among the few ways to diagnose lupus, to distinguish lupus symptoms from other problems, and to
keep this elusive disease in check.

Notes

Tests and procedures are a mirror of lupus activity. Be
sure to ask your doctor about the tests you take. Understanding these procedures—what they tell and how they
turn out—will help you understand your disease better
AND help you take better control of it.

Tests I've Taken	Date	Reason	Result

CHAPTER 3

The Anatomy
of Lupus

"What is happening to my body?"

Knowing that you have a condition called lupus goes only so far to explain the strange and unpredictable symptoms you may experience. The real answer to the persistent question above is found in the very cells of your body, specifically the cells of your immune system.

What follows is a look at what is happening to your body from the inside out. We start with a primer on the healthy immune system and how it goes awry with lupus, and end with an in-depth review of the symptoms of lupus.

The Immune System

The immune system is the body's defense team. It's a network of cells that guard the body against an outside world teeming with potential enemies—bacteria, parasites, viruses, fungi. In one way or another, almost every cell in the body takes part in the defense work of the immune system.

Self vs. Nonself

The wonder of the immune system is its ability to distinguish the "self" from the "nonself"—substances that rightly belong to the body from those that don't. Almost every cell in the body is marked by a molecule that signals "self." This includes cells from every body system— the heart, lung, blood, tissues, et cetera. The healthy immune system knows to leave these marked cells alone.

But anything that isn't a "self" molecule–carrying member of the body catches the attention of the defense team and triggers an immune response. The "nonself" proteins that trigger an immune response are known as **antigens**. The word "antigen" literally means "against a species" ("anti" for against, "gen" for species, kind or type).

Where Is the Immune System?

Stationed throughout the body are organs that breed and nurture the varied members of the immune system's defense team. Known as lymphoid organs, they include

- the tonsils and adenoids
- the lymph nodes
- the thymus
- the spleen

- Peyer's patches
- the appendix
- the bone marrow
- the lymphatic vessels

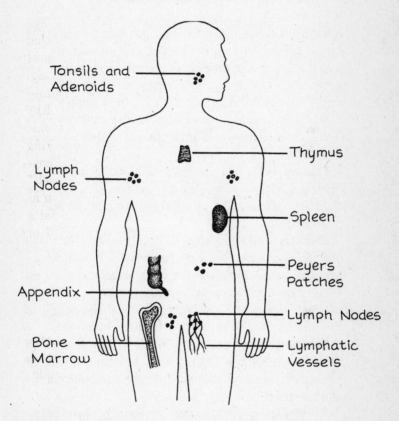

Like all cells, the immune system's defense team is born in the bone marrow. Some of these cells grow up to become **lymphocytes,** while others become **phagocytes**. Immune cells then travel to the immune organs, where they wait for signals to launch an attack against any intruder.

Lymphocytes—Also called lymph cells, lymphocytes are small white blood cells that carry out much of the immune defense. There are three types of lymphocytes: **B cells, T cells** and **natural killer cells**.

- **B cells,** which mature in the bone marrow, are the brains behind antibodies. Each B cell makes only one specific type of antibody, designed to stop and destroy one specific type of antigen. When a B cell comes across an unknown antigen, for example a flu virus, it immediately creates a model antibody. The B cell then clones itself into **plasma cells** and **memory cells**.

  Plasma cells are factories that make millions of identical copies of the model antibody, which are then sent off into the bloodstream to hunt down the offending antigen.

  Memory cells are clones of antibodies. But they are more pumped-up versions of the B cell prototype, and lie in wait for the next antigen onslaught. When the antigen next attacks, memory cells are ready to pounce. Some vaccines take advantage of this mechanism to create, or **induce,** immunity.

  Antibodies are part of a group of proteins called **immunoglobulins (Ig)**. There are nine different classes of immunoglobulins. IgE, for example, causes allergic reactions.

  Antibodies have a varied arsenal in their battle against antigens. They form a deadly bond with the antigen called an **antibody-antigen complex** or an **immune complex**. Antibodies can also coat antigens with a special material that traps other cells that, in turn, engulf and destroy the antigen. Antibodies also block antigen from entering "self" cells.

In most cases, the antibody-antigen complex sets off a chemical reaction involving complement (see below), which ends with the release of toxic enzymes.

Some B cells naturally make antibodies against cells of the self (autoantibodies). In the healthy immune system, suppressor T cells (see below) keep these autoantibodies in check. Part of the problem in lupus, as we'll discuss later, is that the suppressor T cells fail to control the production of these autoantibodies.

- **T cells,** which mature in the thymus (the glandular structure at the base of the neck), are divided into two groups: **regulatory T cells** and **cytotoxic T cells.** Cytotoxic (which means "toxic to cells") T cells directly attack infected or malignant cells.

  Regulatory T cells, sometimes known as helper T cells, are commanders of the B cell army: they activate and suppress them. These cells release **lymphokines,** which, among other things, contribute to the inflammatory response.

- **Natural killer cells** directly attack alien cells by unleashing toxic chemicals.

Phagocytes—These are large white cells which, true to their name, eat ("phago") cells ("cytes") and digest them. Or they trap the antigen and hand it over to B cells or T cells. This group of cell-eaters includes **monocytes, macrophages** and **granulocytes.**

- **Monocytes** and **macrophages** ("mono" means single or one; "macro" means big; "phage" means eater) patrol the blood system for dead cells as well as antigens. Called to action by T cells, these scavengers engulf and present their prey cells to T cells. They also pick the bloodstream clean of antibody-antigen complexes.

- **Granulocytes** are a group of white blood cells including **neutrophils, eosinophils** and **basophils**. These cells have granules, or little capsules, filled with lethal chemicals. Like all phagocytes, the granulocytes engulf antigen. The chemicals in the capsules help them digest these alien invaders.

Complement—The **complement** system is a group of more than twenty proteins which in their effort to control infection contribute to inflammation. The linking of antibody to antigen stimulates a chain reaction of complement. At the end of this chain is a **membrane attack complex**—a kind of sword that punctures the target antigen, causing it to explode.

In people with lupus, levels of complement are lower than normal, either because of the high level of inflammation or because of a disease-related problem in producing it.

Inflammation—In inflammation, complement signals blood vessels to open up wider, ushering in more blood—and defenses—to fight off the antigen. This is what causes the redness of inflammation around an infected area. The macrophages, called to the battle site by T cells, release toxic substances that help them digest immune complexes. (While these substances often help in defense, they can also spill out into healthy tissue and start mistakenly eating away at it, as though it were antigen.) Complement also makes the vessels leaky, allowing white cells to pour into tissue. This is what causes the swelling and tenderness of inflammation.

The end of the immune response—Once the offending antigen is under control, T cells call a halt to the immune reaction. Ending the immune response is just as important as starting it. If the T cells don't signal an end to immune activity, the inflammatory process will continue uncontrolled. As you'll see below, with lupus this overzealous immune reaction can cause direct harm to the body.

How the Team Works Together

The immune response is triggered in two ways. Macrophages jump-start the immune response by trapping antigens, in a process called cell-mediated immunity. This starts one chain reaction. B cells start the immune response by locking on to antigen, in a process called humoral immunity. This starts another chain reaction. Both lines of defense are often activated at the same time.

When the immune response is triggered by macrophages (cell-mediated immunity),

- Macrophages trap and digest antigen.

- T cells attach to macrophages and release lymphokines (enzymes).

- Lymphokines and T cells send out signals to the immune system to create killer T cells and other T cells.

- Killer T cells hunt down and destroy other antigen.

- Once the antigen is under control, suppressor T cells stop the immune system reaction.

When the immune response is triggered by B cells (humoral immunity),

- B cells create antibodies to antigen.

- T cells release lymphokines, which signal the B cells to produce clones.

- B cells clone into plasma cells—factories for antibodies—and memory cells.

- Antibodies, aided by helper T cells, lock on to antigen to form an antibody-antigen complex, or immune complex.

- The antibody-antigen complex triggers a complement reaction.

- The complement chain reaction activates an inflammatory response.

- Small blood vessels swell (dilate) to bring in more blood, creating redness (erythema).

- Vessels become leaky, allowing immune substances to saturate the infected tissue, which creates swelling and tenderness.

- Suppressor T cells call an end to the battle.

- Macrophages consume immune complex debris.

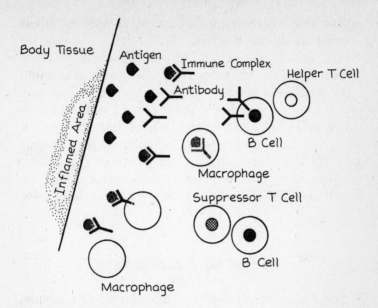

The healthy immune response. *When bacteria, viruses or other antigen get into the bloodstream, helper T cells sound the battle cry. They direct B cells to make antibodies—a perfect interlocking match for the enemy antigen. The antibody-antigen complex, or immune complex, sets off a chain reaction of complement proteins. Complement delivers a lethal blow to the antigen, which triggers inflammation—opening the veins' floodgates for more immune defense. The immune complex is swept out of circulation by macrophages. Once the antigen is under control, suppressor T cells call a halt to antibody production.*

False Alarm: Allergy

There is no biologic reason pollen should bother people. But in some people, the immune system falsely perceives pollen and other benign substances as harmful aliens, causing an allergic reaction.

When an antigen causes an allergic reaction, it's called an **allergen**. On exposure to an allergen, B cells and T cells produce a specific allergy antibody called IgE, which links up with a granulocyte—mast cells (in tissue) or basophils (in blood). From this home base, the IgE antibody is ready to latch on to and trap any passing allergen. The antibody-allergen complex activates the release of chemicals—histamines and others—which cause the symptoms of allergy such as itchy eyes and runny nose.

The Self as Antigen: Lupus

The lupus immune system, like the allergic immune system, suffers from a serious case of myopia. It mistakes the self for nonself. As a result, the immune system attacks the very being it's meant to protect: the self. To put it another way, the body acts as though it were suddenly allergic to its own blood.

The body's own cells, tissues and organs become the innocent targets of antibodies (or autoantibodies, because they're directed against the self). Instead of attacking alien substances, the misguided autoantibodies target healthy cells, cell components and tissue. They react against the fundamental structure of cells—the nuclei (core) of cells and part of the cell walls (phospholipids).

In people with lupus, the immune system falters on several other levels: the B cells are hypercharged and the team of suppressor T cells is understaffed. As a result, not only does the immune system attack the wrong target (cells from its own body), but the immune response gets out of control.

Another major problem is that the antibody-antigen complex, normally swept out of the bloodstream by macrophages, cannot be removed. It lingers and accumulates on tissues. As you remember, the complexes activate complement, which ends in inflammation. In lupus, these immune complexes cause inflammation wherever they settle.

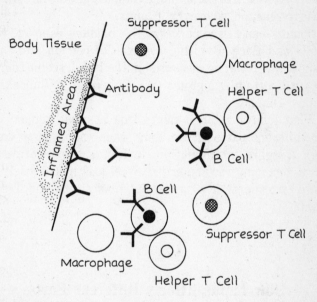

The lupus immune response. *In the lupus immune system, the target antigen is not foreign or harmful: it is the self. B cells make too many antibodies, and suppressor T cells lack the power to control it. Autoantibodies continue to form out of control. Free from the jaws of hungry macrophages, autoantibody-antigen immune complex lodges in tissues. The complement chain reaction causes inflammation wherever complex settles.*

From Cells to Symptoms

It's the inflammation—the end result of the immune reaction—that causes most of the symptoms of lupus. As discussed above, the antibody-antigen complex can find its way to almost any tissue of the body. And like a stray ember from a fire, the immune complex ignites an inflammatory reaction wherever it lands.

Doctors can't predict *where* the immune complex will settle and flare. But the presence of certain autoantibodies, which can be measured in the blood, seems to link up with certain symptoms (see Chapter 2, "Unmasking Lupus: Diagnosis").

What follows is an in-depth look at what happens to the different parts of the body when the immune complex triggers inflammation, including the treatments most commonly recommended. We'll look more closely at these treatments in Chapter 5, "Medications and Treatments."

How Lupus Affects Different Parts of the Body

Lupus and the Joints

Medical term:	Arthritis
Percent of people with lupus who have it:	90 or more. Arthritis-like symptoms are shared by more people with lupus than any other symptom.
Cause:	Inflammation of the joints

Symptoms: Fleeting pain, swelling and tenderness of the fingers, wrists, knees, elbows. Several joints are usually involved at the same time; if only one joint is disturbed or the back feels stiff, it's probably not related to lupus.

Can be confused with: Osteoarthritis or rheumatoid arthritis

How it differs: Lupus arthritis usually does *not* cause long-term damage to the joints. It only rarely results in loss of function or deformity.

Treatment: Nonsteroidal antiinflammatory drugs (NSAIDs) and/or hydroxychloroquine help relieve the inflammation and pain of SLE arthritis in most people. Corticosteroids are seldom needed, and then only in low doses.

                          Exercise is an important part of treatment. A personalized program, based on your own abilities, may be recommended by your doctor.

Lupus and the Muscles

Medical term: Myositis

Cause: Inflammation of the muscles

Percent of people with lupus who have it: 30

Can be confused
   with: Arthritis, flu, muscular dystrophy

Symptoms: Deterioration of the muscles,
                      weakness, pain, tenderness—
                      usually of the neck, shoulder, hip
                      area, upper arms or thighs. The
                      main symptom is weakness, which
                      can be felt as an overall, intense
                      heaviness of the limbs or as a flu-
                      like achiness in which every bone in
                      the body seems to hurt. Because
                      nerves can also be affected by
                      inflammation of the muscles, hands
                      and feet may also feel weak.

Treatment: The aim of treatment is to put a
                      quick stop to inflammation, which is
                      the culprit behind damage to and
                      deterioration of the muscles. For
                      this reason, treatment often starts
                      off with high doses of
                      corticosteroids. Doctors will often
                      keep an eye on progress by
                      measuring enzymes (CPK and
                      aldolase) and slowly lowering the
                      dose until the symptoms disappear
                      and the blood levels of enzymes are
                      normal.

                      Once the inflammation is under
                      control, an exercise program is
                      usually recommended to help keep
                      up muscular strength.

Lupus and the Kidneys

Because kidney (in medical terms, "renal") involvement in lupus is so common, so potentially serious and a bit more complex than other areas, it deserves a closer look.

Each of our two kidneys is reddish brown and about the size of a large bar of soap. At any one time 25 percent of the blood pumped from the heart is coursing through the kidneys. They are an elaborate filtration system; their main job is to purify the blood. They also adjust the volume of blood for a healthy blood pressure and maintain a delicate balance of nutrients and waste. Each day, the kidneys process about 45 gallons of fluid; only about a quart leaves the body as urine.

The kidneys contain about a million microscopic filtering units, called **nephrons**. Each nephron has two main parts. The **glomerulus** is a tuft of filtering capillaries (tiny veins); it's surrounded by a sleeve called **Bowman's capsule**. Bowman's capsule is attached to the **tubule**, which leads the remaining filtered substance, **filtrate**, out of the kidney.

Blood enters the kidney through the renal arteries (the main arteries leading into the kidney). The pressure of the heartbeat forces the blood into the nephrons, and then into the glomerulus.

The vessels in the glomerulus have very thin walls, which helps them perform their main duty as filters. When blood enters, the glomerulus traps larger molecules such as proteins and blood cells. The rest (the filtrate) filters out of the glomerulus and is collected in Bowman's capsule. From here the remaining filtrate goes through another filtering in the tubules, and the remaining waste (urine) is processed through the ureters into the bladder.

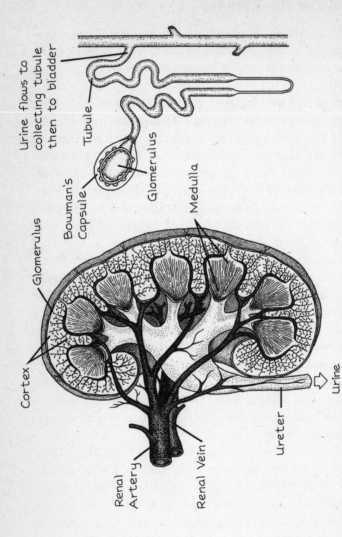

Urine flows to
collecting tubule
then to bladder

Tubule

Bowman's
Capsule

Glomerulus

Glomerulus

Medulla

Cortex

Renal
Artery

Renal Vein

Ureter

Urine

The healthy kidney. *The glomerulus and tubules filter out impurities from the blood. The remaining waste product, urine, empties out of the kidney and into the bladder.*

The knot of tiny vessels that make up the glomerulus creates a perfect trap for large immune complexes. When inflamed, the glomerulus doesn't do its filtering job well; proteins and other waste products escape its fine net and get recycled back into the bloodstream. As these waste products build up, symptoms begin to appear. If the inflammation continues, damage to the nephrons can become permanent and the kidney may stop functioning altogether.

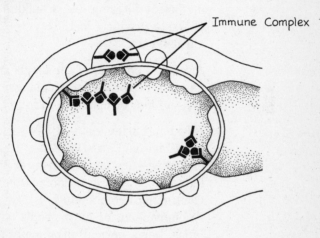

Immune Complex

The kidney with lupus inflammation. *Immune complexes settle in the fine filter of the glomerulus, allowing them to build up in the bloodstream.*

Medical terms:	Nephritis, glomerulitis, glomerulonephritis
Percent of people with lupus who have it:	50
Cause:	Lupus nephritis is defined as inflammation of the nephrons in the

kidneys, the body's filtration system. Lupus glomerulitis is inflammation of the glomerulus. Since most of the body's blood circulates through the kidneys, it makes sense that immune complexes, antibodies and complement will find their way to these organs, causing inflammation, inefficient filtering and a buildup of waste products in the bloodstream.

Symptoms:

Swelling **(edema)** of the hands and feet, water retention, weight gain, nausea, loss of appetite, fatigue

Pattern:

Blood and urine tests—BUN serum creatinine and creatinine clearance—are used to monitor the kidney for signs of inflammation. Continuing urine analysis is recommended for most people with lupus, but a normal urine analysis may not show kidney problems. Kidney biopsy is the most accurate way of tracking renal function.

Treatment:

Treatment is first aimed at controlling the problems resulting from nephritis, such as high blood pressure and fluid imbalances.

Milder forms of the disease usually require little or no treatment with corticosteroids. But more severe cases may need corticosteroids.

There are several ways
corticosteroids may be given.

Alternate-day oral therapy, which
means taking the drug by mouth
every other day, has proved useful
in people who have kidney disease
only; those with other symptoms
may need the continuing control of
daily therapy.

Pulse therapy, or high doses given
by injection for several days in a
row at regular intervals (for
example, once a month), is
prescribed by some doctors for
people whose nephritis has rapidly
become worse.

Immunosuppressive drugs kill
cells and calm down the immune
system. They are often used in
cancer chemotherapy. Taken either
alone or in combination with
corticosteroids, immunosuppressive
drugs are sometimes used in more
advanced cases of nephritis or
glomerulitis.

Hemodialysis is a procedure
wherein the blood is passed through
an artificial filter; it's usually
reserved for people with rapid
decline of kidney function.

Plasmapheresis involves drawing
blood and removing the immune

complexes from the plasma, then
returning healthy cells to the body.

In some cases, the kidney fails
despite all measures. In these rare
situations, continuing hemodialysis
may be necessary to support kidney
function. Alternately, **peritoneal
dialysis** may be used. In this
procedure the body's own
abdominal cavity serves as the
filter, and fluid is drained out of a
catheter. With such treatment,
some people recover enough
function to stop using the artificial
dialysis either completely or at
least for a while. **Kidney
transplant** techniques have also
improved so much in recent years
that transplant has become a viable
option for many people with chronic
kidney failure.

It's generally recommended that
people with severe nephritis avoid
aspirin and other nonsteroidal
antiinflammatory drugs (NSAIDs)
such as ibuprofen because they may
cause additional injury to the
kidney.

Lupus and the Heart

Medical terms:	Pericarditis (inflammation of the lining of the heart), myocarditis (inflammation of the heart muscle), coronary artery disease (blockage of arteries), arteritis (inflammation of the arteries)
Causes:	See Medical Terms
Percent of people with lupus who have it:	20 to 30
Symptoms:	Pericarditis: fever, chest pain, fast heartbeat; coronary artery disease: chest pain (angina); myocarditis: irregular heartbeat, shortness of breath
Treatment:	For pericarditis, inflammation is usually treated with low doses of corticosteroids or NSAIDs. Coronary artery disease may occur in people with lupus as an adverse effect of corticosteroid therapy, which is known to cause high cholesterol, blood clots and blockage of the arteries. As a result, corticosteroids are not usually recommended and treatment depends on the individual. Myocarditis is much less common, but it can be life-threatening and usually requires hospitalization and high doses of corticosteroids.

Lupus and Infection

Causes:

People with lupus seem to be more prone to infection than the general population. There are a few possible reasons. First, corticosteroids and immunosuppressive (cytotoxic) drugs are known to increase the risk of infection by inhibiting the body's defense mechanisms. Scientists have also proved that lupus causes a defect in the body's ability to kill bacteria and viruses. The types of infections vary widely, including those caused by bacteria and viruses.

Percent of people with lupus who have it:

about 85

Symptoms:

Fever, sweats, chills and pain are the most common symptoms. Infections tend to focus in the lung, skin and urinary tract.

Treatment:

Treatment is the same for people with lupus as it is for others, using a wide range of antimicrobial drugs specific to the bacteria, fungus or virus that's causing the infection. For example, an infection caused by the bacteria *Staphylococcus* would require an antibiotic designed to kill those particular microbes. Similarly, a yeast infection calls for drugs that kill yeast organisms. There is a notable exception: sulfa-based antibiotics should be avoided because they tend to exacerbate lupus symptoms, and may even provoke flares.

Lupus and the Lungs

Lung involvement with lupus can take several different forms. The most common is **pleurisy,** or **pleuritis** (described below)—inflammation of the lining of the lung. But there are other ways the lung can suffer from lupus inflammation. **Chronic lupus pneumonia (pneumonitis)** is caused by inflammation and fibrosis, or scarring. The symptoms start out with a dry cough and shortness of breath that can slowly worsen. Mild cases don't require treatment, while severe cases may require corticosteroids or immunosuppressive drugs. **Acute lupus pneumonitis** afflicts up to 15 percent of people with lupus. Symptoms are fever, shortness of breath, chest pains and cough that produces mucus or blood. **Pulmonary hypertension** is rare. It's caused by inflammation and deposits of immune complexes on the arteries that lead to the lung. Shortness of breath and heart failure are the symptoms. Also rare is **pulmonary hemorrhage,** which produces shortness of breath and the coughing up of blood. This severe condition may necessitate the use of a ventilator and/or treatment with immunosuppressive drugs and corticosteroids. Plasmapheresis, which filters out the immune complexes, may also help people with hemorrhage. People taking immunosuppressive drugs may be more prone to **pulmonary infections** because of the lower resistance to bacteria.

Medical terms:	Pleuritis, pleurisy
Cause:	Inflammation of the lining of the lung
Percent of people with lupus who have it:	30 to 60
Symptoms:	Chest pain on taking a deep breath, and a dry cough. (Coughing blood or mucus, with fever, is probably a sign of pneumonia, a complication of immunosuppressive drugs, which requires a different type of treatment than pleuritis.) Some people may have fluid in the lung lining, or **pleural effusion**.
Treatment:	NSAIDs are usually recommended for pleuritis. Low doses of corticosteroids may be needed if there is also a pleural effusion.

Lupus and the Blood

Medical terms:	Anemia (low red cell count), thrombocytopenia (low platelet count), granulocytopenia and lymphopenia (low white blood cell count)
Causes:	There are several possible causes for anemia: autoantibodies against red cells may form, causing **hemolytic anemia,** a condition in which red cells die prematurely; chronic inflammation can lower

production of red cells; and anemia may also be a by-product of kidney problems or chronic blood loss (ulcers, heavy menstruation).

When antibodies attack platelets, the condition is called **immune thrombocytopenia (ITP)**. Granulocytopenia and lymphocytopenia result either from autoantibodies or a sensitivity to certain medicines.

Percent of people with lupus who have it:

50

Symptoms:

Fatigue is the main symptom of anemia. Thrombocytopenia may show up as easy bruising, tiny red dots on the skin or bleeding from the gums or nose. Granulocytopenia and lymphocytopenia rarely cause symptoms you can see or feel.

Treatment:

The treatment for anemia depends on the cause. For hemolytic anemia or anemia caused by chronic inflammation, corticosteroids are the first choice; if this fails, then the spleen may need to be removed. In anemia caused by kidney disease, male hormones or, rarely, blood transfusions may be called for. Anemia caused by blood loss often responds to iron supplements, as well as correction of the blood loss.

When thrombocytopenia is caused
by autoantibodies against platelets
(immune thrombocytopenia),
corticosteroids are first
recommended.

In granulocytopenia and lymphocytopenia, there are usually no symptoms, so treatment is rarely needed.

Lupus and the Blood Vessels

Medical term: Vasculitis

Cause: Inflammation of the blood vessels—
                       capillaries (tiny vessels), arterioles
                       (medium-sized vessels) and arteries
                       (large vessels)—caused by deposits
                       of immune complexes on the vessel
                       walls. In severe cases, the result is
                       destruction of the vessel wall and
                       blockage of the vessel.

Percent of people
  with lupus who
  have it: Not known

Symptoms: Blood vessels thread throughout
                       the body; the symptoms of
                       vasculitis depend on the location of
                       the vessels. For example, if the
                       vessels leading to the hand are
                       affected, symptoms may appear in
                       the hand. Below are some of the
                       more common ways vasculitis may
                       show itself in a person with lupus:

Constitutional (body-wide):
fever, achiness, weight loss and
fatigue
Joints: Achiness, arthritis-like
swelling and pain
Kidneys (rare): high blood
pressure
Intestines: cramps, bloating and, in
severe cases where gangrene
occurs, blood in the stools
Skin: small red dots on legs
(petechiae), larger dots (purpura),
large bruises; more rarely, hives
and rashes and small black spots at
the end of fingers and toes (nail fold
infarcts) or gangrene
Eyes: Visual blurring or loss of
some vision
Heart (rare): chest pain
Lung: coughing, fever and, rarely,
shortness of breath caused by
scarring of lung tissue

Treatment:

Therapy depends on the location of
the problem: doctors will want to
treat the immediate problem as
well as the underlying cause
(inflammation). For inflammation,
corticosteroids are usually the first
choice; if this fails,
immunosuppressive drugs are
sometimes used. Plasmapheresis—
rinsing the blood free of immune
complexes—may be recommended
in rare cases.

Lupus and the Brain

Medical terms:	Cerebritis, central nervous system (CNS) lupus
Cause:	Not completely understood, but cerebritis may be caused by autoantibodies against tissue of the brain or nervous system. Distinguishing true disease from emotional problems related to having lupus can be a challenge for both the doctor and the person with lupus.
Percent of people with lupus who have it:	Up to 50
Symptoms:	The symptoms vary widely in cerebritis, but can be divided into three categories: physical (organic) emotional and psychiatric.

The symptoms vary widely in cerebritis, but can be divided into three categories: physical (organic) emotional and psychiatric.

Most often the symptoms are mild, including headache, dizziness or vision problems. More severe—and rarer—symptoms include seizures, stroke, acute psychosis and a host of other neurologic and psychologic problems.

Very often people have trouble coping with lupus, suffering depression, anxiety or other emotional problems, but this does not mean lupus has affected the brain. It's up to your doctor to conduct the proper tests to rule out a physical cause for your symptoms. We'll look at the emotional aspects of having lupus in the next chapter.

Treatment:

Before prescribing treatment, it's extremely important to find the cause of symptoms: do they stem from physical disease **(organic symptoms)** or emotional conflicts **(somatic symptoms)**? If they're not emotional, are the symptoms caused by lupus or another problem? A series of tests, possibly including a CAT scan or an EEG (see Chapter 2) may be needed to answer these questions.

Psychological and nervous system problems caused by lupus respond very well to corticosteroids. Seizures may also require specific medication, such as anticonvulsants. Anxiety and depression also demand their own unique approach; a combination of counseling and drug therapy may be called for.

Other Conditions Related to Lupus

Skin symptoms take different forms. Some people get a redness across the nose and cheeks in the shape of a butterfly, known as the butterfly rash or malar rash ("mala" means jawbone or cheek in Latin). Another type of skin reaction is a raised, bumpy red rash, sometimes triggered by exposure to the sun. These eruptions can easily be confused with hives, allergies or psoriasis. Usually they appear on the face or scalp.

Lupus can produce small bumps, like cysts, under the skin, which are sometimes confused with rheumatoid arthritis. Bruises are more common in people with lupus who also have a low platelet count.

Ulcers in the mouth and nasal passages can occur; they may or may not be painful.

Discoid lupus—red, scaly, disc-shaped patches—can create serious cosmetic problems. The lesions start out small, but can grow larger and spread. In about 50 percent of people with discoid lupus, the sun seems to make the problem worse. These lesions will go away with time, but they may leave behind broken blood vessels, scars, darker or lighter skin and, if the scalp is involved, bald spots.

Fewer than 10 percent of people with discoid lupus go on to have systemic lupus. But up to 15 percent of people with systemic lupus have discoid lupus.

Tiredness is one of the most persistent and draining symptoms of lupus. Unlike the everyday fatigue of living a full life, the lupus fatigue can be heavy and all-consuming. Feeling "bone-tired" can be a warning sign of a flare.

People with lupus have more than their fair share of **fevers**—either long, drawn-out periods of low-grade fever or a sudden spike in temperature. These feverish periods may signal a flare or an infection.

Urinary tract infections (UTI) seem more common in people with lupus, for various reasons. First, women as a group are more prone to UTI, and lupus is a disease of women. Also, the disease process impairs the ability to fight off infection. Finally, corticosteroids and other medications for lupus often predispose a person to infections.

Raynaud's disease is a condition that people with lupus as well as people without lupus suffer. In lupus, it may herald a milder course of disease. Its hallmarks are a change in color—to red, white or blue—in the fingers, the toes and sometimes the nose and ears. Cold temperatures may cause a tingling sensation. Raynaud's is caused by an extreme sensitivity to temperature and treated by taking preventive measures: wearing gloves in the cold, keeping uncovered hands out of the freezer and, in some cases, taking drugs that open up the blood vessels.

Sjogren's syndrome is an autoimmune disease that occurs in people with lupus (and related diseases). It causes dry eyes and mouth due to inflammation of the salivary glands and lacrimal (tear) glands. Some people may suffer arthritis symptoms, pain and stiffness, dry skin or rashes. Treatment aims to return moisture to the eyes and mouth. The patient may be told to use artificial tears and humidifiers and to drink plenty of fluids.

Scleroderma has received a lot of attention lately as an adverse effect of breast implants. It's an autoimmune disease whose symptoms start out like those of Raynaud's disease and lead to swelling of the fingers and toes. Arthritis pain, muscle weakness and tightening of the skin may occur. Symptoms can extend throughout the body, including tissue scarring in the lungs, heart and intestines. Treatment aims to reduce inflammation, pain and the immune response.

An Important Note

We would hate to end this chapter leaving readers burdened with the long, exhausting list of lupus symptoms. We cannot overemphasize that most people with lupus do not suffer from severe disease—that's a rarity. It's also important to know that symptoms come and go. Very seldom do people with lupus live in continuous pain.

CHAPTER 4

Emotional Trials and Triumphs

Few things are certain in life, and there are even fewer certainties when your life includes lupus. The unpredictable pattern of flares creates the perfect breeding ground for emotional confusion. In fact, it's safe to say that the emotional effects of lupus need just as much attention as the physical problems. In this chapter, we'll review some of the ways lupus can upset your emotional balance—and strategies for regaining it.

Though we've tried to cover most of the emotional issues that come up, they deserve more attention than this book allows. Other authors have explored them in more depth. We urge you to investigate some of the thoughtful, helpful texts listed in the "Resources" section at the end of this book.

Your Style of Coping

How do you cope with life's stresses? By denying them? Overreacting to them? Asking for help? Expect an exaggerated reaction to the stresses of coping with a chronic disease like lupus. Half the battle in conquering lupus is overcoming emotional stumbling blocks. We're not talking about psychological symptoms caused by the disease, such as cerebritis, but the emotional burden of facing a lifetime with lupus.

Now is the time to break away from old coping strategies that don't work and to replace them with approaches that do. The first step is knowing the areas that need changing.

Fighting Through Fears and Anxieties

Who doesn't feel afraid at one time or another? Fear is a basic instinct that serves a function, protecting us and keeping us from acting recklessly. Without a healthy dose of fear, we might not avoid oncoming traffic, or turn at a strange noise.

But when you have lupus, there seems so much more to be afraid of. You may fear not being believed. Before your diagnosis, when your symptoms were a mystery, doctors and loved ones may have been skeptical. The longer the disease remained unnamed, the more your self-doubt may have grown—along with your mistrust of others. By the time you received a diagnosis, mistrust may have become a habit, one that distanced you from others.

Even after your diagnosis, friends and family may have

a hard time grasping the scope of your suffering. Lupus so often wears a mask of health: friends exclaim that you look just fine when you're suffering from numbing fatigue, muscle weakness or pain. The dual nature of lupus can take a heavy toll on your confidence. For many of us, a feeling of helplessness surfaces when we perceive that calls for aid fall on deaf ears.

This helpless feeling may feed already existing anxieties that lupus will flare, that it will shift to another part of the body, or that it will leave you more disabled and dependent.

Your fear may be more vague, focused on an unknown something out there that will do you harm—the way lupus has done. Or your fear may be very specific. Many people fear the loss of relationships with people who don't understand—or accept—their disease. Many women fear passing lupus on to their children. Other concerns revolve around the ability to work.

Are these fears healthy or unhealthy? The answer depends on how you react.

Facing and Erasing Your Fears

Why is it so important to face your fears? If you're like most people, you may not be aware of your fears and the way they drive your actions. We mostly fear the unknown; like the imaginary monster in the closet, we fear the worst when we don't confront it. If left in their hiding places, fearful attitudes control us, sometimes preventing us from fulfilling our goals. But when faced head-on, the pure facts we learn about lupus can be real fear-busters. When confronted, our concerns can even inspire positive action.

For example, your anxieties about lupus flares may

lead you to take better care of your body, to avoid situations that trigger flares (see Chapter 6, "Preventing a Flare") and to take medications as prescribed. You may read more books about lupus, speak with your doctor about your concerns, get involved with lupus support groups. The learning and interaction shed light on the dark mystery of disease, defuse fears and empower you with a better sense of control.

Some people react to fear by drawing closer to others. If you're not embarrassed by your fear, you may find comfort in sharing your experiences and feelings with family and friends. In doing so, you strengthen your bonds with these loved ones. Sharing fears with others who have lupus often uncovers solutions to anxieties—especially when they have to do with practical issues, such as the workplace, parenthood and daily tasks. Lupus support-group meetings are wonderful places for picking up ways of coping with the limitations of the disease.

On the other hand, some people give in to their fears and make drastic changes in their lives. Left unchecked, fears become phobias. Some people may give up traveling lest a flare leave them stranded without medication or medical care. Others take their fear to the extreme and never leave their homes. In their attempt to control their disease, they let lupus control them.

Or they may allow the fear to well up inside, unspoken. Instead of sharing concerns with family, friends and doctors, they withdraw. They may feel that facing these fears is too painful—or that it might be too painful for others to share. The result is a self-imposed isolation that may eventually wear away at relationships. Depression (discussed below) is a common by-product of repressed fears and isolation.

This is not to judge, or to dismiss the fear of a recurrence: this fear is one of the greater challenges facing people with lupus. And overcoming it takes a strong effort, starting with facing fear head-on. Your fears may be your own creation, but that doesn't mean you have to conquer them alone. Most of us need help untangling these confusing emotions. Family, friends, support groups and your doctor are there for just that reason.

Also, to some degree, the cliché holds true: time is a great healer. If you were just recently diagnosed, your body has suddenly become a mystery. Your life patterns are changing every day. You may need to relearn your body. It may not happen overnight: allow yourself the time you need. Remember, you don't have to solve the problems of lupus *this minute*. In time, you'll pick up practical ways to dodge a flare (see Chapter 6). You'll begin to see that your body can bounce back from a flare. You'll start to accept certain limitations and work around them, rather than let them stop you from living your life to its fullest. You'll tune in to your body's new needs and learn how to meet them. Just give yourself a chance.

Turning Anger Around

From our earliest years, many of us are taught that anger is negative and inappropriate. We're generally expected to express our thoughts rationally, to face adversity with wisdom and positive solutions.

If our society is unskilled at accepting anger, we're even less nimble at handling it. Like the hot potato, no one wants to be caught with anger. In our culture, there's something almost shameful about admitting to irrational feelings like anger. As a result, when life deals us an unexpected blow, few of us are emotionally prepared to fight back—even though that may be our natural instinct.

But is anger really so irrational? If you're combating lupus (rather than submitting to it), isn't it logical to rally a fighting spirit? And unless you're vying for sainthood, isn't it normal to feel frustrated when disease suddenly dive-bombs into your life and disrupts your plans or goals—whether caring for your children, going to parties or finishing a project?

Far from being shameful or irrational, anger is a normal response to having lupus. The problem is, how do you express anger so that it doesn't infect and inhibit your life or alienate those you love? With lupus, expressing anger can pose a problem. If someone does you wrong, you know where to aim your anger. You can release it by telling that person off. As long as you don't hurt that person or yourself, expressing your anger is a pretty effective way of letting it go. But with lupus, the cause is unknown. No single person or thing owns the blame. As a result, your anger can easily become misdirected—toward the doctor who diagnosed you, toward your family and friends for not understanding or supporting you enough, or toward yourself.

Understanding Anger

Resentment, rage and indignation are three ways people express anger, according to psychologist Robert H. Phillips in *Coping with Lupus*.

Does your anger smolder beneath a cheerful facade? You may resent events or people (including yourself). Resentment is anger unresolved. You'll know you're resentful if you often have negative feelings about a person but never express your reasons for feeling angry. Your resentment may come out as little jabs against that person, or as neglect. For example, you may resent the fact that your friends, who are more active than you, don't always include you in their activities. Rationally, you may know that they're trying to protect you and that it's not really fair to be angry with them, but you feel angry anyway. As a result, you may be a little cooler toward them than usual. Perhaps you're oversensitive, reading negative meanings into innocent remarks.

Do you find yourself responding explosively to frustrations? Rage may be your mode of expressing anger. Rage is a lot easier to recognize than resentment, but it's not necessarily easier to control. Getting to the real source of anger is one way to cut the fuse on explosive anger. If you see red when your kids leave the den a mess, are you really angry at them, or are you ticked off at yourself for letting things get out of control? Take a look at what makes you angry, why, and how you can better express it next time (see the anger-releasing exercises below).

If you can express your anger clearly, in a controlled and rational way, congratulations. Indignation, the "healthy" way of expressing anger, may be your anger-releasing method. But even well-controlled anger can get out of hand if it's your response to too many situations—or if it's expressed in a belittling way.

After you've recognized your anger, it's important to find the cause. For people with lupus, the anger-triggering scenarios are many and diverse. Friends and family may seem to expect too much, insensitively asking you for favors that would wear you out. Your kids may not help enough around the house. On the other hand, loved ones may coddle you too much, making you feel incapable and confirming your own fears about being left helpless by lupus.

You may also feel anger at friends and family for not

really accepting your illness. How many times have you heard people tell you how good you look? Though intended as a compliment, it may sound as if they're trying to deny your illness. The implicit message seems to be "You can't be very sick if you look so good."

Feelings of victimization are second cousins to anger. With no one to blame, we often turn on ourselves, or feel self-blame and self-pity. "Why me? What did I do to deserve this fate?" are common questions that lead to self-blame. And self-blame is a dead end. As far as lupus experts know, there's nothing a person can do to prevent lupus. So how can you be held responsible for it?

As with fear and many other emotions, anger is a natural response. In itself, it's neither healthy nor unhealthy. It all depends on how you cope with it.

Anger-Releasing Exercises

The first step toward dealing with anger is acknowledging it. Make a list of the people and situations that make you angry. Don't judge your anger. Let yourself go completely.

If you're having a hard time getting your feelings down, try this exercise: with pen and paper handy, set a kitchen timer for fifteen minutes. For a title, put down "What Makes Me Angry About Having Lupus." Then start writing. The only rule is that you must not stop writing until the timer goes off. If you hit a stumbling block, write about whatever crosses your mind. Just keep that pen in motion.

Once your list is made, take a serious look at it. Again, don't judge; accept your anger and focus on *why* these things make you angry. This may not erase your anger, but it may help you see it in a clearer light. Peggy Maddox, author of *On the Edge: Health Crisis, Helping Yourself* offers seven practical steps for channeling anger:

1. Cry. When you're angry, you can feel like a boiling kettle bursting to whistle. Crying or screaming into a pillow can offer some much-needed physical release for pent-up anger.

2. Strike out at something. Punch a pillow or a mattress. Go to a gym and sock a punching bag.

3. Vent positively. Anger is a form of power—a positive form when it's vented in a positive way. Write a letter to your congressional representatives asking them to support research funds for treatment of lupus, or write to the FDA to ask for more aid toward cures for less acknowledged diseases such as lupus. Write to the American Medical Association for more information about experimental drugs. Join your local Lupus Foundation (see "Resources") to get more information about the disease, to learn more ways to promote the cause of lupus research and cure, and to discover ways you help other people with lupus deal with their problems.

4. Record your feelings. Write them down; talk into a tape recorder. According to Maddox, expressing anger is the first step toward releasing it. You're not locked into holding these angry feelings—when you've written them down and feel ready, try tearing up the paper.

5. Schedule your anger. Rather than let your anger permeate your life, make an appointment to deal with it. Write your angry feelings down and schedule fifteen minutes in the day to deal with them. If anger insists on intruding outside your "anger hours," jot your feelings down and force yourself to put them aside until the appointed time.

6. Love yourself. Maddox contends that most anger is directed against the self. To counteract this, don't delay writing down your best attributes. Start right now with a list of what makes you uniquely wonderful. It sounds corny and self-absorbed, but who will know but you? And the results may help you to release some self-blame.

7. Talk with others. By sharing your concerns with friends, family, counselors, religious leaders or support groups, you not only gain a new perspective on your problem, but you may also help others understand theirs. (Adapted from *"On the Edge: Health Crisis, Helping Yourself"* by Peggy Maddox, published by Glenbridge Publishing, Limited, 1991. Used by permission.)

As a final word on anger, remember that your goal is to *express* your feelings. It's a bonus if you can actually change the situation that's making you angry. If you find yourself forever dissatisfied, *you* are responsible for finding a different way of changing that. How many times can you tell someone you're upset? How long can you resent having lupus? If the situation doesn't change, you must change your approach.

And remember: anger is a very powerful emotion. If you have the power to be angry, you have the power to change an unhappy situation—or at least your way of handling it.

Dealing with Depression

Though each of us feels depressed at some time in our life, chronic illness seems to make us more prone to depression. According to some experts, the average person takes two years to adjust emotionally to having lupus. During this adjustment period, the physical ups and downs of lupus can take the emotions on a roller-coaster ride—a quick route to depression.

Unlike fear or anger, depression is often a hybrid of feelings. A profound sadness, a feeling of helplessness and of being out of control, fear of what the future will bring, guilt and self-blame about the past, lack of self-esteem—these are just a few feelings that can breed depression.

In people with lupus, depression may be triggered by a single event or an accumulation of events. Many of us have a hard time accepting the chronic nature of lupus: knowing that lupus can't be cured or that we may depend on medication for the rest of our lives can make the future look bleak. Our body image and self-confidence (and relationships) can suffer deeply from cosmetic changes, pain and disability.

Having lupus may mean a change in lifestyle and relationships. Unable to be as physically active as before, especially in our favorite activities, we may feel deprived and depressed. Our life's path may be rerouted by the limitations of having lupus. Being unable to measure up to our expectations, or the expectations of others, can leave us feeling emotionally at odds. For example, you may feel unworthy and sad because you can no longer care for your family the way you could before. Or you may feel that your skin reactions will make you unattractive.

Like fear, anger and anxiety, depression is also a natural response to chronic illness. Similar to a period of mourning, depression can be a time to feel, express and grieve for the loss of your pre-lupus lifestyle. But it's important to know *why* you feel a certain way. You may need to go through a short period of sadness to take a new step in understanding your illness and accepting your new life. Once you see the cause of your conflicting feelings, you have a starting point for solving them. The

key phrase here is "short period." Left on its own, depression can breed more depression, beginning a down-
ward spiral that can even cause physical problems.

When does depression become an emotional problem
that needs attention? Doctors who study depression face
this challenge in all types of patients. What follows is a
discussion of some warning signs of serious depression—
signs that should lead you to seek help.

When to Worry About Depression

More than a long period of the blues, depression means
a sense of despair that seems to seep into all daily activities. We don't sleep well—either too little or too heavily.
During waking hours, we're anxious and restless, or le-
thargic and uninterested. Even things that used to make
us happy bring us little joy. Concentration becomes difficult and our mental faculties slip. Seemingly for no reason, we tend to cry more often. Depression leaves people
without hope that their symptoms will ever go away.
Others may feel helpless, thinking that no one cares
enough to help them, or that they'll fail if they try.

Depression is such a powerful disease that it doesn't
just affect the mind, but often afflicts the body. In fact,
doctors looking for signs of depression often examine the
body. But this presents a problem because the physical
symptoms of depression can resemble lupus symptoms.
Fatigue, lethargy, pain and headache are common physical features of depression that can be confused with lupus. Other ways in which the body expresses depression
include loss of sexual drive, indigestion and other minor
ailments.

How can anyone ignore weeks or months of despon-
dency? Unfortunately, long bouts of depression are often

ignored—by doctors as well as their depressed patients. Even families may tend to explain depression away as a natural response to having lupus, not realizing that depression doesn't have to be a constant companion to disease. And, when confronted by their changes in behavior, depressed people often deny their negative feelings.

If you recognize symptoms of depression in yourself or a loved one, it's important to acknowledge them and to know that depression is highly treatable. Most people respond well to treatment, whether a short course of medication or counseling, or both.

Defeating Depression

Robert Phillips recommends a dual strategy for battling depression: "Get thoughtful and get physical." Start out by making a list of the things that depress you. Then divide the list into two more: the things you can change and the things you can't. Act on the things on the first list, and change your thinking about the things on the second list. If you're depressed about not being able to throw a big party this New Year's Eve, that goes in the first list, "Things I Can Change." Feeling depressed about the fact that you have lupus goes in the second list, "Things I Can't Change." Let's look at both of these as examples.

You want to throw a big party for New Year's Eve, but you know it will just wear you out. You become very depressed, not so much because you can't have the party, but because it's symbolic of all the things you enjoy that you can't do because of lupus. First step: express your feelings. Before your disappointment and anger snowball into a full-blown depression, try to talk them out with a friend. Not only will you feel better for having released some of these pent-up feelings, but your friend may even offer some alternatives. Next step: consider what you'll miss most about the New Year's Eve bash. If you can't have the whole thing, try to capture the essence that gives you the most joy. Instead of a big party, try a small get-together, or a potluck.

There are a few messages here:

- Look within and face the feelings causing your depression. Don't let your sad feelings run away with your life. Make a list of reasons you're unhappy. Try to figure out when you're most susceptible to these feelings.

- Take a realistic look at your abilities—and your limitations. Then ensure success by making your goals reachable. Schedule one appointment instead of four; have a potluck instead of a big dinner party; start a car pool instead of shuttling your kids around every day. But do make plans. Make lists for the day and check tasks off as you accomplish them.

- Stop comparing yourself now to yourself before. In many ways, lupus means a new start in life—a life that's different from the one you had before. Is this change necessarily bad? It may seem so if you compare it to your pre-lupus life. Your new life may be slower than the one you had before. But the new pace may give you a chance to see and experience things you once missed. Maybe you can start enjoying hobbies that match your abilities. Instead of seeing this change as a liability, try to experience it as an opportunity.

- Get creative. How creative can you be with your life now that you have lupus? The way you answer this question will determine the quality of your life.

When you stop to think of it, this is the challenge that faces all of us in life—whether or not we have a chronic disease. A successful life is one that's lived to its fullest potential. You can't expect more from yourself than that.

- Gather your network of support. Whom can you count on? Who can't handle your illness? I'm not suggesting that you cut ties with those unable to give you support. They may change over time (other people need to adjust to your illness, too!). But focus on those who are there for you.

Above all, know that depression can be lifted. Get help—from your doctor, friends, family, from local lupus support groups. Have faith in the willingness and ability of others to help.

A Word About Sharing with Others

When lupus appears in your life, its effects will ripple throughout your support system. Your family may go through as many emotional trials as you do. Your friends may not know how to react. They may overreact, smothering you with attention instead of really communicating with you. In short, friends and family may not always be able to listen when you need to let out your feelings. You'll learn who in your circle can handle a close account of your feelings, and who can't. Some of your friends simply need time to adjust, just as you do. Others may never adjust. What does this mean? Choose your confidants with care. You want a listener who can be there for you, and you don't want to pressure someone who can't. But also accept that even the closest friend or family member may falter in the role of confidant and pillar of strength.

You can also expect family life to go through some changes. The alteration in your role may shift the way everyone else interacts. Prior problems may come forth with more force under the stress of dealing with these changes.

In a way, support groups offer the ideal outlet. Lupus support groups exist in every state of the union (see "Resources"). If there isn't a lupus group near you, consider other types of support groups, such as those for people with chronic illness or with arthritis (if you suffer from arthritis-like symptoms).

Finally, you may need counseling by a professional experienced in dealing with chronic illness.

We'll discuss some of the ways lupus affects relationships later in this chapter.

The Way We See Ourselves

Lupus not only changes the way we look at the world, it can also change the way we see ourselves.

Socially . . .

In some cases, your physical appearance changes. Skin reactions may cause rashes and marks, some of which leave scars, or hair loss. Mouth and nose ulcers may break out. These problems can pose a short-term or a chronic cosmetic dilemma. In some people, high doses of corticosteroids cause weight gain, bloating and a "moon face."

Lupus pain and fatigue can also deliver a blow to your self-image. Suddenly you're playing mild-mannered observer instead of your former superenergetic, do-it-all self. The emotions that result—frustration, anger, fear, self-pity—become partners to pain. For example: you have a big event coming up, and no matter how much you rest, you still feel tired. The stress and anxiety that result may cause your muscles to tense, which increases the intensity of pain and fatigue. The more pain and fatigue you feel, the more depressed and frustrated. A vicious cycle results.

Some people withdraw from social activities for fear of the way others will perceive them. Insecurity is infectious: self-consciousness about your appearance may spread to other areas of life, causing you to shy away from activities even after the rash has disappeared.

To stop the cycle, isolate the problem. If your self-image is suffering from a change in your appearance, do your best to improve it. You deserve to lavish time and attention on yourself, whether by changing your hairstyle, buying flattering clothing, or just making the effort to eat sensibly.

To some degree, the physical symptoms of lupus can be treated (see Chapter 5) or avoided (see Chapter 6). But flares may happen nonetheless—and they may come at the least welcome of times, such as before a big event. In fact, they may be more likely to appear in times of stress. What then? Makeup (water-based), hats and other accessories can do wonders to improve a seemingly disastrous cosmetic problem. Dazzling earrings serve as handy diversions from a small mouth ulcer. If the cosmetic problem can't be camouflaged, it's up to you how brave you want to be.

Physical pain and fatigue wear away at self-esteem more subtly. While cosmetic flares come and go, physical limitations can change the way we see our place in the world in a more permanent way. It may not be easy to accept that you can't do as much as before, but instead of focusing on what you can't do, focus on what you can. Then shape your goals to match your abilities. Set yourself up for success, not failure.

Romantically and Sexually . . .

Lower self-esteem can also affect your love life. Even in times of the best health, all relationships need maintenance. When one partner goes through changes, the couple changes, and must adapt. Chronic illness can put even the most stable relationship to the test. As much as your partner may understand your need for more rest on some days, feelings of guilt, resentment or fear may arise—in both of you.

And then there's sex. Though lupus never affects the genitals, we all know that sex is tied up with our mental well-being and our self-image—and sexuality can be shaken by lupus. Perhaps you feel self-conscious and less attractive, which can definitely affect the libido. Your partner may be less sexually assertive, thinking you need rest, when in fact you want to make love. Or you may be sending "stay away" signals because you feel unattractive, but you really want your partner to come closer. The possibilities for mixed messages are almost endless.

While sex may not be the most important part of a relationship, it does deserve special attention. Open communications are an absolute must. This is not a time to be reclusive. While withdrawal may be a normal reaction to a damaged self-image, it's not a helpful one. Just as it's important to face anger, fear and depression, it's vital to break out of the withdrawal cycle.

But how? With honesty and all the love you feel for that person. Without trust, no relationship is worth a hill of beans. Summon all the trust you have for your partner and let him or her know how you feel. Remember, if you can't have the torrid sex life you once did, that doesn't mean you have to let the fires go completely cold. Affection is a good way to kindle a warm glow.

On the purely practical level, there are ways to make sex more comfortable. Robert Phillips recommends the following:

- If you suffer joint pain, limber up for sex. Do a few stretching exercises to help your body get in the mood.

- If you suffer from the chilliness of Raynaud's disease, try a warm bath and raise the temperature in the bedroom.

- If you have oral or vaginal ulcers, get treatment. Though they may be painful, these ulcers are not contagious.

- If you have vaginal dryness due to Sjogren's syndrome, it may take you longer to become lubricated. So take it slow. Or try a vaginal lubricant, but make sure it's water-soluble.

- Whatever your problem, experiment with different positions. Readjusting your sex life need not be a chore!

- If your self-esteem is bruised, indulge yourself a little. Take some time to make yourself look and feel better.

New love relationships pose a different set of concerns. How do you tell a new love interest you have lupus? The

answer is, with sensitivity. As with anyone you tell, remember that few people have an accurate understanding
of lupus. It's up to you to anticipate, and preempt, their
concerns. Let your new partner know that lupus is not
contagious and is rarely passed on from parent to child.
See Chapter 1, "Lupus Lore vs. Reality," for some more
facts about lupus. But as important as the facts are your
feelings. Let your new friend in on some of your feelings.
It's one way for him or her to learn about you.

Parenting Problems and Solutions

Lupus may take lots of things away from you, but it
can't touch what children need most: your love. This is
especially true for younger children. So whatever the
challenges that lie ahead, keep in mind that your love is
always there and that it's the most important thing you
can give.

Helping Kids Cope

As your children age, the issues can become more complicated. Your bouts with flares can leave them fearing
loss: of your time together, of the security of a "normal"
family life, and perhaps most profoundly, the loss of your
life.

In keeping with our credo that honesty is the best pol-
icy, your children should learn as much about your condition as they can understand. It's hard for children to
grasp that you don't always have the energy to play or
go to Little League games or school parties, or even to
drive them around. That's why it's important to take time

to talk. Help them understand that there are times when you can't be available because of your illness, but you still love them. It's equally important to assure your children that you're not going to die.

Even though you can't be the do-everything mom or dad, you can still spend time with your children. Set aside regular special times together. You can enjoy a quiet activity that doesn't demand a lot of energy, like doing puzzles, reading out loud or just talking. It doesn't have to be a long period, either.

Adolescence is a trying stage even when a parent doesn't have a chronic illness. But dealing with a parent who's "different" from others, or a household routine with extra responsibilities, or a family at odds because of the stresses of disease, adds another dimension to the generation gap. When striking out on their own and carving their own identity is their biggest desire, your teens may feel guilty about wanting to spend less time at home. They may resent the burdens of added family chores. Or they may harbor deep fears about losing you, at the same time they want to separate from you.

What's a parent to do? Let your teenagers be your guide. What are their main concerns? What are their difficulties in dealing with your condition—or with life in general? Struggling between childhood and adulthood, they may need extra reassurance. Or it may be time to start approaching them like adults. While they may not be ready for the full spectrum of your emotions, your children may respond well to your invitations to express theirs. If you expect them to shoulder more responsibilities, Dr. Phillips recommends you allow them more adult privileges.

Parenting Without Guilt

Lupus can put a heavy guilt trip on parents. Your physical limitations during flares may leave you less able to perform normal duties or even to play with your children. Feelings of guilt and inadequacy can compound the stresses of illness. Your resentments about lupus may extend to your kids or spouse when they fail to do their share of housework. All these feelings can create a big knot of emotions.

Keep the lines of communication open. What is making you feel guilty? Angry? Try to understand your feelings, then express them to your family. If you feel guilty, let them know. They might not mind having take-out pizza instead of homemade dinners a few times a week—they might even like it. If you feel angry, pinpoint the reasons and let them out clearly (the key word is "clearly"). Ask them to help you with solutions. But before you express your feelings, it's important to try to understand them yourself. See the earlier sections for some pointers on dealing with anger, fear and depression.

Dealing with Doctors

Doctors can be the objects of intense emotions. After all, they're the ones who delivered the bad news. They send you from test to test. They give you medications, some of which have uncomfortable effects. Many of your feelings and confusions about lupus can easily be projected onto your doctor. Unlike many other relationships, the one you have with your doctor can determine your physical health. It's especially important to be honest here and let your doctor know how you're feeling—both physically and emotionally. This is often easier said than done.

Lots of people become tongue-tied when they go to the doctor. They leave frustrated because they forgot to mention this symptom or that one. They leave angry because the doctor didn't ask certain questions or pick up on hints.

Take some control over your health—and help your doctor help you. Between visits, keep a running list of symptoms and concerns. These could be physical symptoms or questions about medications. (If you have side effects, don't delay: call your doctor immediately.) Organize your notes before your next visit. Write them down (use the worksheet below) and give the doctor a copy. If you still have questions after you leave, call back. With a condition as complicated, subtle, changeable and elusive as lupus, you must be flexible with your doctor.

Practical Pointers for Communicating with Your Doctor

- Make a list of questions *before* your visit. Don't be shy about referring to the list, and writing down the answers, while you're with your doctor.

- Feel free to phone. If you leave the office with questions, don't dismiss them. Give the office a call. If the doctor can't help you right away, maybe another staff member can.

- Face your fears. You're probably imagining the worst—you may have a problem that's easily resolved. But you won't know unless you speak up.

- Accept your embarrassment. Tell the doctor if the subject is hard for you to discuss. Don't be afraid to ask for sympathy and help.

- Insist on concerned, considerate treatment. If you aren't happy with the way your doctor responds to you, say so. If necessary, find another doctor.

- Get the facts straight. Watch out for outdated and false information. Ask for literature and other educational materials your doctor can provide to help you understand your problem and its treatment.

Office Visit Worksheet

Use this worksheet to help organize your thoughts before visiting your doctor.

Symptoms   Date

_____

_____

_____

_____

_____

_____

Medications/reactions

_____

_____

_____

_____

_____

Other issues

_____

_____

_____

_____

_____

_____

_____

_____

_____

_____

_____

_____

_____

_____

_____

_____

PART II

Coping with Lupus

Taking Action

Now that we've looked at the story behind lupus—the who, what and why of the disease—let's shift our attention to action. What can you do to lessen its effects on your body? How can you live with lupus? You may feel discouraged to hear that there's no cure for lupus. But remember: even though there's no miracle drug or vaccine (yet), you're not helpless. Far from it. There are lots of things you can do to live a healthier life with lupus. And you can start today.

In this segment of the book, we'll home in on different strategies for living with lupus. By strategies I mean a combination of options that together create a treatment plan. Your strategy could include medications, diet, exercise or all three. We'll examine each of these options individually—which we hope will expand your vocabulary for discussing them with your doctor.

In Chapter 5, we'll review medications commonly used to calm or prevent flares. You'll learn how the drugs work (as far as that's known), the side effects some people experience (and how to ease some of them) and drug interactions to beware of.

By now you know that flares are caused by inflammation of tissues. What you may not know is that flares can sometimes be predicted—and avoided. In other words, where there's fire, there's often smoke. In Chapter 6, we'll review the common "smoke signals" of an upcoming flare and efforts you can make to avoid it entirely, or at least prevent it from worsening. This chapter will also make you aware of events in your life that cause flares, such as stress and sun exposure.

Women make up 90 percent of the people with lupus, and most are in their childbearing years. Pregnancy is naturally an issue of great concern. In Chapter 7, you'll learn how pregnancy can affect lupus—and how lupus may affect pregnancy. More importantly, you'll pick up some pointers for a healthy pregnancy and delivery.

There's no evidence that diet or exercise can alter the immune problems that cause lupus. But following certain guidelines may help relieve some symptoms of the disease or ease side effects of certain medications. In Chapter 8, we'll show you how.

We'll also look into the future of lupus research and treatment. Are scientists uncovering clues to the cause of lupus? Which new treatments are being tested? Find out in Chapter 9.

Our knowledge about lupus grows almost daily. To help you keep up to date, we provide resources at the end of this book. Through the organizations and publications listed, you can get firsthand information about the latest in lupus research and treatment. Through local chapters of the Lupus Foundation of America, you'll discover that you're not alone. Thousands of women and men across the country face challenges similar to yours. Lupus may not be the most common disease, but the support network is vast and able. You'll only find out how much it can help by calling. And who knows? Your experiences might be of great value to someone else with lupus.

CHAPTER 5

Medications and Treatments

Creating a treatment plan for a person with lupus is like putting together a puzzle. Your symptoms, your general health, your age and your lifestyle are pieces of a bigger picture that together define your treatment needs. For this reason, it's next to impossible to expect general guidelines to work for every person with lupus. Each person reading this book is unique and deserves individual care. Only someone with an intimate knowledge of your symptoms and your lifestyle—like your doctor—can make useful, safe recommendations.

With that said, it's natural to wonder about the value of this chapter on medications and treatments. The reason for this chapter is simple: if you understand how and why a drug works, you may feel more confident about taking it. And when you take a drug as prescribed, you increase your chances of getting the desired effect (as long as you're not allergic to it or otherwise sensitive). For example, many people think drugs for lupus just relieve symptoms. But with lupus, it's important to know that most recommended drugs do more than cover up the problem and make you feel better; some drugs actually interfere with the disease process. Perfect examples are the NSAIDs (nonsteroidal antiinflammatory drugs), such as ibuprofen and aspirin. You may be used to taking these drugs for aches and pains, knowing that they're not necessarily helping the *cause* of those aches and pains. You may also think that because they're not prescription drugs, NSAIDs aren't really important. But for people with lupus, NSAIDs do more than relieve pain. They can stop a flare in its tracks by reducing inflammation—an important goal, as you know.

Side effects are another reason it's wise to know about medications and treatments. Every action has a reaction. With drugs, sometimes the reaction isn't always healthy or comfortable. For example, while helping to stop inflammation or busting up immune complexes, antimalarial drugs may also negatively affect other parts of the body. An unpleasant or unhealthy response to a drug given at the recommended dose is called an adverse effect. This is different from a toxic reaction or overdose, which comes from taking too much of a drug.

It's easy to blame lupus for most types of discomfort when in fact "symptoms" may be caused by the drugs used to treat the disease. On the other hand, the so-called side effects may really be symptoms. Either way, you need to keep in close touch with your doctor about any reactions while you're taking medicine.

When you suspect that the side effects are caused by drugs, it's tempting just to stop taking the drug—or take less of it. Don't: let your doctor know first. There are real health risks involved in playing around with dosages of medications. For example, abrupt changes in corticosteroid doses—either increases or decreases—can cause severe and permanent damage. So talk to your doctor.

How can he or she give you good care if you don't speak
up when you have questions, problems or pain?

As you've probably figured out by reading Chapter 3,
treatment is often determined by symptoms and by their
location in your body. The severity of the problem may
also influence the treatment. Table 4 outlines common
problems with lupus and the treatments commonly given
for these problems, discussing each drug individually.

Table 4. Common Lupus Symptoms and Treatments

Symptom	Drug Treatment Option(s)
Joints Arthritis	NSAIDs Hydroxychloroquine
Muscles Myositis	Corticosteroids
Kidneys Nephritis	Corticosteroids —Alternate-day therapy —Pulse therapy
Severe nephritis	Immunosuppressive drugs Hemodialysis Plasmapheresis Total nodal radiation
Kidney failure	Hemodialysis Peritoneal dialysis Kidney transplant
Heart Pericarditis, myocarditis	Corticosteroids

Lungs

Pleuritis	NSAIDs
	Corticosteroids

Chronic lupus pneumonia/
pneumonitis

—Mild	No treatment
—Severe	Corticosteroids
	Immunosuppressive drugs

Acute lupus pneumonitis	Corticosteroids

Pulmonary hemorrhage	Intravenous steroids
	Immunosuppressive drugs
	Plasmapheresis

Pulmonary hypertension	Corticosteroids

Lazy/elevated diaphragm	Corticosteroids

Blood

Anemia	Corticosteroids
—Severe hemolysis	Removal of the spleen
—Secondary to kidney disease	Hormone therapy (erythropoietin)
	Blood transfusions
—Caused by blood loss	Transfusion

Thrombocytopenia	Corticosteroids

Blood vessels

Vasculitis	Corticosteroids
—If corticosteroids fail	Immunosuppressive drugs
—In rare cases	Plasmapheresis

Brain

Cerebritis

—Psychological expressions	Corticosteroids

—Seizures	Corticosteroids
	Anticonvulsants
—Anxiety	Corticosteroids
	Anxiolytics
	Counseling
—Depression	Corticosteroids
	Antidepressants
	Counseling

Skin

Discoid lupus	Antimalarial drugs
	Topical corticosteroids
Subacute cutaneous lupus erythematosus	Antimalarial drugs
	Topical corticosteroids

Eyes and mouth

Sjogren's syndrome	Humidifier
—Dry eyes	Artificial tears
—Dry mouth	
Mouth ulcers	Topical anaesthetics
	Topical corticosteroids

After you read this chapter, we hope you'll understand why your doctor recommended a certain treatment, the types of side effects commonly (and uncommonly) experienced with that treatment and some ways you can cope with them.

Nonsteroidal Antiinflammatory Drugs (NSAIDs)

Don't be put off by this long word. It's a fancy term for a class of drugs that includes that old familiar medicine-cabinet standby, aspirin. As the name clearly says, NSAIDs are antiinflammatory drugs. The name also tells us that they aren't steroids (*non*steroidal). Why does the name tell you what the drug *isn't?* The answer is that corticosteroids are the classic antiinflammatory drug, and they are in a class by themselves. NSAIDs are antiinflammatory drugs of a different sort—they work in a completely different way from corticosteroids.

Not all NSAIDs are alike. There are aspirin-like NSAIDs, which are called salicylates. Then there are NSAIDs different from aspirin, including ibuprofen (brand names Motrin and Nuprin), naproxen (brand name Naprosen) and sulindac (brand name Clinoril). Some of the NSAIDs are longer-acting than others; some are more expensive; others may be more conducive to unwanted interactions with other drugs.

How NSAIDs Work

Aspirin and most other NSAIDs are painkillers. They block the sensation of pain by acting on the nervous system. But at higher doses, many of them also can stop inflammation. How? As you learned in Chapter 3, inflammation doesn't just happen all at once; it's the end result of a chain of chemical actions and reactions. Prostaglandins are natural chemicals in the body that help ("mediate") the inflammatory process. NSAIDs block prostaglandins from forming and in this way cut off the inflammatory process. Some researchers think NSAIDs also help calm the immune system by calling suppressor T cells to action. (You may remember that part of the problem with the lupus immune system may be that T cells are in short supply. As a result, the immune system and inflammation rampage out of control. By summoning more T cells, NSAIDs may help overcome this glitch in the immune system.)

Your doctor and you are the best judges of the dose that's right for you. The product package offers general guidelines for the doses usually prescribed for pain and inflammation. The right dose is usually based on your size (weight and height), your age and your physical health. So consult with your doctor for the correct dosage for you.

Adverse Effects

The common problems with NSAIDs occur in the gastrointestinal (GI) tract (stomach upset, heartburn, diarrhea), the kidney and the blood platelets. Why do these problems happen? Remember that prostaglandin is a natural chemical, an essential step in inflammation. It also helps protect cells and tissues. By blocking prostaglandins, NSAIDs help stop inflammation—and may also leave certain tissues vulnerable to breakdown.

The lining of the stomach is especially vulnerable to NSAIDs. This makes sense, since NSAIDs have to travel through the GI tract before becoming available to the body at large. Gastric ulcers can occur—without any painful symptoms—early on in therapy. Diarrhea and stomach upset can also cause discomfort to people taking NSAIDs.

To help prevent the adverse gastric effects of NSAIDs, some doctors recommend adding misoprostil, a prostaglandin-like drug. The idea is to squash inflammation with the NSAID and prevent tissue breakdown with the extra prostaglandin. This new strategy seems to lower the risk of gastric ulcer, but the long-term effects of misoprostil aren't yet known.

Some people who take a lot of NSAIDs may experience blood thinning: it may take the blood platelets longer than normal to form blood clots. This effect, along with a higher risk of bleeding, ulcers and bruising, is easier to manage with non-aspirinlike NSAIDs. For this reason, patients should stop taking NSAIDs for a period well before and after any surgery.

Aspirin may cause nervous system effects, such as ringing in the ears. This side effect may be a toxicity, a sign that you're taking too much aspirin. Let your doctor know.

Easing NSAIDs' Side Effects

To ease the stomach upset, take NSAIDs with food. Also, ask your doctor about different types of formulations, such as enteric coated aspirin, which may be easier to swallow. It may require some give and take and experimentation—under your doctor's guidance—to find the dose and the formulation that work right for you.

Be wary of NSAIDs if you have a low platelet count or other clotting problems. Also, those of you with kidney involvement should be very wary of NSAIDs, as they may lower the blood flow to your kidneys. Not all NSAIDs have this effect, so consult your doctor first.

Don't take the drug if you've had an allergic reaction to it before, if you have a peptic ulcer, if you have impaired liver function or if you have high blood pressure or a history of heart failure.

Antimalarials

Quinine, the grandfather of modern antimalarial drugs, comes from the bark of a Peruvian tree. It wasn't until seventy years after its discovery that quinine served lupus patients in treating skin lesions. Today, derivatives of quinine—chloroquine (brand name Aralen), quinacrine (brand name Atabrine) and hydroxychloroquine (brand name Plaquenil)—are the most commonly used for lupus. Hydroxychloroquine is more popular because it seems to have fewer side effects.

Antimalarials are mostly used to treat ultraviolet light–related skin symptoms (SLE, discoid lupus and subcutaneous lupus), joint symptoms, pleurisy and lupus fatigue. Some researchers have shown that continuous antimalarial therapy prevents flares. Antimalarials also come to the aid of people with other lupus-related immune disorders. They're prescribed alone, or teamed up with corticosteroids or aspirin. It's believed that antimalarials can help lower the necessary dose of corticosteroids.

How (We Think) Antimalarials Work

After more than a century of use, researchers still don't know exactly why antimalarials help people with lupus, but they have some good leads. Antimalarials block prostaglandins, inhibit immune complexes and absorb ultraviolet light—just three reasons these drugs may be useful in lupus.

Adverse Effects

With antimalarials, the risk of adverse effects is linked closely to the dose: the higher the dose, the more likely an adverse effect. Other than their bitter taste, though, side effects are pretty rare with antimalarials. (A coated formulation has recently become available that makes antimalarials easier to swallow.) Stomach upset is the most common side effect of all antimalarials. Some people taking quinacrine may experience a yellowing of the skin, eyes and urine. With long-term use, quinacrine or chloroquine may also cause blue-black discoloration of the palate or nails, as well as loss of hearing. Chloroquine may cause premature graying or loss of hair, but it's rare. But with long-term treatment, all antimalarials can accumulate in the retina and, rarely, cause damage to the retina and cornea, and blindness. Damage to the cornea is often preceded by a loss of feeling in the eye or blurred vision.

Coping with Antimalarial Therapy

There are a few ways that you can avoid the vision-damaging side effects of antimalarials. The trick is to catch any damage—and discontinue the drug—as early as possible. Since damage may occur without changes in vision, it's critical to get tested regularly. An ophthalmologist should examine your eyes every six months, starting before treatment begins. Some doctors recommend that patients take an Amsler grid test regularly. The Amsler grid is a sheet of paper, like graph paper, filled with small squares. If you notice a fuzziness or wavering when you look at the paper it may be an early sign of eye damage.

Avoid antimalarials if you are pregnant, or want to become pregnant, unless there are no other options. Consult your physician about the issue. Also, you should not take antimalarials if you have liver disease, bone marrow disease or a blood disorder.

Corticosteroids

Corticosteroids landed in the lives of people with lupus like a "scientific bombshell," in the words of one early scientist. They changed the reputation of lupus from a fatal disease to a chronic, manageable disorder. They gave new life to people with lupus.

Much is known about why corticosteroids work in reducing lupus inflammation. They're the most potent antiinflammatory drugs available. And if you've read the previous chapters, you know that inflammation is the disabling feature of lupus.

You'll hear corticosteroids referred to also as prednisone, glucocorticoids, adrenocorticoids and steroids (though they shouldn't be confused with the bodybuilding steroids). Corticosteroids are all related to a natural hormone called cortisol, which is produced in the body by the adrenal glands. It's vital to many life-supporting functions. Cortisol helps the body metabolize fats, carbohydrates and other nutrients. Our bodies can't survive without cortisol. People with lupus need more cortisol than the body makes naturally because of the overactive immune system and the overabundance of inflammation.

Cortisone was the first manufactured corticosteroid; prednisone, prednilosone and other drugs are chemically similar to corticosteroids. They can be taken in pills, in cream or ointment, or by injection.

How the Body Makes Cortisol

The body naturally makes cortisol by a network of interacting systems called the HPA axis. The **hypo-thalamus** stimulates the **pituitary glands**, which stimulate the **adrenal glands** to make cortisol. The body pumps up cortisol production under stressful conditions—illness, injury or severe emotional upset. If the stress continues for a long period and cortisol levels in the body get high enough, the body will start to think it has enough cortisol and will stop producing it. This is called negative feedback. The same negative feedback happens with synthetic cortisol, such as prednisone. Prednisone floods the system, fooling the body into believing it's making enough cortisol. The adrenal glands start to shrink because the body no longer needs to make cortisol. As a result, the body becomes dependent on the artificial prednisone. *This body change is why it's dangerous to stop taking prednisone abruptly.* You must taper off and give the body a chance to start making cortisol itself. Let your doctor make dosage changes.

How Corticosteroids Work

Corticosteroids douse inflammation from a few directions. They stop neutrophils from reaching the tissue. T cells and B cells (which make antibodies) become scarce. Also, corticosteroids block interleukin-1, which plays a role in immune cell interactions and in fever.

As a result of their multipronged action, corticosteroids are highly powerful antilupus drugs that can be used for a wide range of symptoms.

Adverse Effects of Corticosteroids

Unfortunately, some people pay a price for the benefits of corticosteroids. As a general rule, the higher the dose, the more severe the reaction. Also, the longer you take corticosteroids, even at low doses, the greater the risk of adverse effects.

Adverse effects can be separated into short-term and long-term. Remember: you won't have all these adverse effects—you may have none—and everyone has a different response.

The short-term effects of corticosteroids are reversible. They'll go away after you stop taking the drug. Also, major, noticeable effects are more likely at higher doses.

Swelling is the most common short-term effect. The drug could cause "moon face" or swollen cheeks, bloating of the stomach and a hump on the back made of adipose tissue. None of these effects is permanent. They all disappear after you stop taking the drug.

Other short-term effects occur in the digestive system. Some people will have an increased appetite, resulting in unwanted weight gain. Heartburn is a problem for others.

Emotions may become unbalanced from cortisone. Some people feel charged up; others get insomnia. Changes in mood—either elation or depression—are not unusual.

Because of their effects on the inflammatory and immune processes, corticosteroids may make you more prone to infections and fevers. The hormonal changes can make menstrual cycles go haywire, or make them stop.

The long-term adverse effects of corticosteroids only occur after long periods of taking the drugs. They are generally more serious than the short-term effects, and efforts are usually made to prevent them by adjusting the dose.

Outer body changes include stretch marks and excessive hair growth. Both, unfortunately, are permanent. You may also notice that you bruise more easily and that you don't heal as quickly; these effects end when you stop taking the drug.

Bone-related problems are potentially quite serious. Osteoporosis is the loss of bone tissue, possibly resulting in fragile bones and a higher likelihood of fracture. Osteonecrosis (damaged bone) afflicts people after long-term treatment with corticosteroids. It usually affects a hip bone.

Arteriosclerosis—narrowing of the vessels leading to the heart—is another serious long-term adverse effect of corticosteroids, one that can result in higher risk of heart attack. High blood pressure is another heart-related problem with corticosteroids. Cataracts (cloudiness of the lens of the eye) may require surgery.

Since corticosteroids affect the body—almost every body system can be touched by corticosteroid treatment—it makes sense that they change the outcome of laboratory tests. Blood glucose, cholesterol, potassium, uric acid and salt levels may rise; calcium and thyroid levels may fall.

When Corticosteroids Are Needed

Your doctor will evaluate the severity of your disease to determine whether or not you need corticosteroids. In people with so-called mild disease—a condition that isn't life-threatening, such as fever, arthritis, rash or tiredness—corticosteroids are only used after less potent (and less risky) medications fail.

For example, if you have fever or joint pain, your doctor may first recommend an NSAID. If that doesn't work, he or she may suggest a different NSAID formulation, then an antimalarial. If that fails, corticosteroids may be prescribed. With rashes and other skin-related conditions, antimalarials can also be used along with corticosteroids.

On the other hand, severe or life-threatening disease conditions can't wait for a trial of less potent drugs. Kidney nephritis, anemia, nervous system involvement, vasculitis and myocarditis are a few conditions that warrant going straight to corticosteroids.

How Doses of Corticosteroids Are Determined

The dose of corticosteroids is highly individual. It's based on your size, your general health and your tolerance of the drug. Doctors usually strive to find the threshold dose—the dose that's tolerable but keeps symptoms from flaring. But in general, the more severe the disease, the higher the dose.

What's a high dose? What's a low dose? Here's how doctors break it down:

High dose: 41 to 120 milligrams per day
Moderate dose: 16–40 milligrams per day
Low dose: less than 15 milligrams per day

In severe disease, a high dose is first given to knock out the inflammation before it causes any permanent damage. Once the inflammation is under control, the corticosteroid dose can be reduced slowly.

Alternate-day therapy—Now that you've read about the adverse effects and possible permanent effects of long-term therapy, you can see why many doctors are reluctant to keep their patients on corticosteroids for long periods. To limit adverse effects, some doctors recommend alternate-day therapy. As the name implies, this means taking corticosteroids every other day instead of each day. In this way, the patient gets the antiinflammatory effect with fewer of the side effects.

Doctors aren't in complete agreement about who is best suited for alternate-day therapy, but most agree that it's most useful in people who need long-term treatment (such as those with kidney problems). It's less appropriate for people with symptoms in more than one part of the body. Most people with multisystem disease need at least daily doses to keep the flare in check; those with fever might even need to take their doses twice a day.

Pulse therapy—In an attempt to lessen the side effects that come with long-term corticosteroid dosing, doctors sometimes try pulse therapy. In this approach, corticosteroids are injected for a few days in a row, but for only a few days a month.

Abruptly lowering corticosteroids can be dangerous. As mentioned above, the body stops making cortisol and becomes dependent on the synthetic corticosteroid. So lowering the corticosteroid dose should be done by tapering off your daily regimen. Let your doctor be your guide.

To lower the corticosteroid dose, some doctors like to compensate with NSAIDs or antimalarials (see p. 124). This approach is called corticosteroid sparing. These drugs boost the antiinflammatory action while lowering the dose—and risks—of corticosteroids.

Corticosteroids also come in a topical form (applied to the skin) for use on lesions. Symptoms are fewer with the topical form, but these creams and ointments are still very potent drugs with the ability to cause serious side effects.

Coping with Corticosteroids

Corticosteroids are powerful drugs and should be taken seriously. It's probably wise to wear a Medic-Alert bracelet in case of an emergency; it's important for doctors to know that you're taking corticosteroids when making decisions about your health.

In your day-to-day life, there are several things you can do to help counteract the negative effects of corticosteroids. Watch your diet carefully. Avoid salt and caffeine to reduce the water-retaining effect of corticosteroids; this will help minimize bloating and limit the probability of high blood pressure.

Since long-term therapy with corticosteroids can weaken bones, talk to your doctor about the pros and cons of taking calcium supplements.

Also, if you're planning to have surgery or dental procedures, remember to let your surgeon or dentist know that you're taking corticosteroids and ask that your physician be contacted.

Immunosuppressive Drugs

In the treatment of potentially serious diseases such as lupus, doctors like to have a trump card up their sleeves for times when all else fails. The immunosuppressives today serve that role. As a "rescue" strategy with some hefty side effects, immunosuppressives are not prescribed lightly. Drugs in this class include cyclophosphamide (brand names Cytoxan and Procytox), azathioprine (brand name Imuran) and cyclosporine (brand name Sandimmune).

Also known as chemotherapy drugs, the immunosuppressives are also used as anticancer drugs. In lupus, they're mostly used for severe, life-threatening conditions such as lupus nephritis, cerebritis, thrombocytopenia, hemolytic anemia, pulmonary hemorrhage and vasculitis.

Often they're used in a corticosteroid-sparing strategy—taken along with corticosteroids so that doses of both drugs can be lowered. In fact, some doctors believe that immunosuppressives are useful only in combination with corticosteroids.

How Immunosuppressives Work

As the name implies, these drugs suppress (calm down) the immune system. You may remember from earlier chapters that lupus inflammation results from an overactive immune system: the body produces too many antibodies against the wrong target (the body's own tissue).

Immunosuppressives are known as cytotoxic agents, meaning they destroy cells. They suppress the immune system by blocking the production of the B cells that make antibodies and suppressing live B cells. They also reduce the levels of some autoantibodies to DNA. The higher the dose, the greater their immunosuppressive effects.

Doses of Immunosuppressives

These drugs are given orally or by injection. Dosage is based on body weight and changed depending on symptoms, blood counts and inflammation. The dose is either taken daily by mouth, or monthly by injection (pulse therapy). Therapy can continue for extended periods—as long as it takes to reduce inflammation.

Adverse Effects

Immunosuppressives are very powerful drugs. They can cause minor problems such as nausea, vomiting and hair loss—or more severe effects.

The severe effects of oral or injected immunosuppressives are of greater concern. They can cause bladder problems, including bleeding ("hemmorhagic cystitis"). Usually the cystitis subsides after a few days. But if it continues for long periods, it may require treatment or transfusions. Blood in the urine, painful urination, swollen feet or pain in the stomach or joints may be a sign of bladder problems.

It's ironic that drugs used to treat cancer—as immunosuppressives are—can also cause cancer. Bladder cancer, blood malignancy and skin cancer are all possible results of long-term therapy with high cumulative doses (a cumulative dose is the total amount of drugs used for therapy from beginning to end of treatment). About half of bladder cancers are curable.

Most immunosuppressives can also have a negative effect on fertility for both men and women who take the drugs for more than a year. Men who take these drugs may have lower sperm counts. Women may suffer fibrosis of the ovary and failure of the ovary. Since the ovary makes estrogen, women experience side effects of estrogen loss, such as hot flashes, osteoporosis, tenderness of vaginal tissue and cessation of periods. If you miss a period, be sure to contact your doctor.

Other side effects include a higher risk of infection (viral and bacterial), interference with healing, congestive heart failure and anemia. Low white blood cell counts and low platelet counts can occur in some patients; both usually appear along with anemia. Shortness of breath or palpitations may be a sign of heart problems; fevers and chills may indicate an infection; a tendency to bleed or bruise more easily may mean a reduction in platelets or white blood cells. Any of these symptoms should be reported to your physician.

Be wary of immunosuppressives if you have irreversible kidney or liver failure, kidney stones or gout, or low white blood cells or platelets. If you are pregnant, most immunosuppressives can cause birth defects and spontaneous abortions. Azathiaprine may not have this effect. Since the final word is not out about the effects of these agents in pregnant women, it's wise to ask your doctor about the latest research.

Taking immunosuppressives can cause irregular results of certain tests, like the candida skin test, the mumps test and the Pap test.

Coping with Immunosuppressives

Some of the milder side effects, such as nausea, can be eased by taking the drug in the morning. Also, your diet can help you deal with the stomach upset. Try eating a light snack before treatment. Instead of having two or three large meals, consider lots of small meals. Eat slowly and chew thoroughly—this aids digestion. Also, avoid drinking with meals.

When taking more than one medication, even if it is not a prescription, you may have a drug interaction. Let your doctor know about any drugs that you are taking.

Table 5. Common Drug Interactions

Drugs	Interact With	May Cause
Antimalarials		
Chloroquine	Penicillamine	Higher risk of penicillamine toxicity
	Magnesium salts	Less chloroquine effect
	Antacids	Less chloroquine effect
Hydroxychloroquine	Same as Chloroquine, plus:	
	Digoxin	Higher risk of digoxin toxicity
Quinacrine	Primaquine	Higher risk of primaquine toxicity
NSAIDs		
	Anticoagulants	Higher risk of bleeding
	Dipyridamole	Higher risk of bleeding
	Indomethacin	Higher risk of bleeding
	Sulfinpyrazone	Higher risk of bleeding
	Valproic acid	Higher risk of bleeding
Indomethacin	Same as NSAIDs, plus:	
	Lithium	Lithium toxicity
	Beta blocker drugs	Less beta blocker effect

	Bumetadine	Less bumetadine effect
	Captopril	Less captopril effect
	Ethacrynic acid	Less ethacrynic acid effect
	Furosemide	Less furosemide effect
Aspirin	Heparin	Higher risk of bleeding
	Methotrexate	Methotrexate toxicity
	Valproic acid	Valproic acid toxicity
Corticosteroids		
	Nicotine	Greater corticosteroid effect
	Isoniazid	Less isoniazid effect
	Aspirin	Less aspirin effect
	Oral anticoagulants	Less or greater anticoagulant effect
	Barbiturates	Less corticosteroid effect
	Phenytoin	Less corticosteroid effect
	Rifampin	Less corticosteroid effect
Cyclophosphamide		
	Allopurinol	Greater bone marrow suppression
Azathioprine	Allopurinol	Greater bone marrow suppression

Plasmapheresis

Plasmapheresis is not a medicine; it's a procedure that involves sifting out antibodies and immune complexes. A

unit of blood is withdrawn and siphoned into a cell sepa-
rator, which removes plasma and red blood cells. The
plasma, which houses the immune complexes and autoantibodies, is put away and the red cells are returned to the
body. This procedure lasts a few hours and carries little
risk. Though plasmapheresis doesn't work for everyone,
it has proved especially useful in people with severe disease who are also taking medications.

Medication Control Checklist

It's not always easy to keep track of medications, especially if you're taking more than one. To get the most out
of them, gather all the information you can. Here's a
checklist of questions to ask your doctor or pharmacist
about the medicines you take.

Name of drug

_____

Is there a less expensive generic form available?

_____

Is the generic equivalent to the brand-name drug?

_____

What is my dose?

_____

What should I avoid while taking this drug (sunlight, driving, certain foods, etc.)?

_____

_____

_____

How should I take this drug?
  —How often?_____
  —With meals/without meals?_____
  —How long will I need to take it?_____

Will any of the drugs I now take affect this new drug? (List drugs you take regularly or might take at some point. Don't forget antacids for heartburn, aspirin, diet pills, vitamins, cough medicine—they all count.)

_____

_____

_____

_____

_____

_____

_____

_____

_____

_____

CHAPTER 6

Preventing a Flare

They say an ounce of prevention is worth a pound of cure. If this adage is true, then people with lupus are in luck, because even though there's no cure for lupus, there are lots of ways to prevent a lupus flare. And when you prevent a flare, you control lupus. There are two keys to preventing flares: avoiding activities that trigger them and recognizing the signs of an upcoming flare.

We already know that a flare results from an autoimmune reaction. While no one is quite sure what inspires the immune system to attack healthy tissue, medical experts have drawn a bead on factors that get the immune system riled up. From scientific studies and reports by people with lupus, experts have identified three potential triggers: ultraviolet (UV) light rays, stress and certain drugs.

In this chapter, you'll learn why certain types of light, stress and medications might send your immune system into flare mode. You'll also learn how to read early warning signals of a flare. Recognizing these signals gives you a head start on treating the flare—and a better chance of extinguishing it.

An Important Lesson in Light

As a source of light, life and warmth, there are few images more positive than the sun. But for many people with lupus, the sun is anything but wholesome: it's a fireball threatening to ignite a flare. When Henrietta Aladjem, lupus educator, activist and author, titled one of her books *The Sun Is My Enemy,* she wasn't just being poetic. As many as 60 percent of people with systemic lupus react to the ultraviolet (UV) light of the sun with flares; the proportion climbs as high as 75 percent among people with discoid lupus. This effect is medically known as **photosensitivity** ("photo" means "light"; photosensitivity is sensitivity to light).

Not everyone with lupus is photosensitive. Some of you will never react to the sun. In rare instances, people go along for years without a problem and suddenly have a reaction. So just because you're not photosensitive now doesn't mean you're immune forever.

Who is most likely to be photosensitive? Of people with systemic lupus who have been studied, white women seem to be most vulnerable, followed by black women, black men and Hispanic women. (Though white men, Asian women and Asian men are less prone to sun-sensitivity, they're not excluded.) People with active disease tend to be more sensitive to UV rays. Those with subacute cutaneous lupus, neonatal lupus or complement deficiency are also more at risk of suffering from UV light.

Many people experience a lag of a few days or weeks between exposure and emergence of symptoms. Skin reactions range from a sunburn-like redness to aggravation of existing lesions to new lesions. But in a person with systemic disease, a rash may come first, followed by body-wide symptoms such as fever, fatigue and flu-like pains—or whatever systemic symptoms are typical of that person.

Know Your UVA's, B's and C's

Photosensitivity is caused by ultraviolet (UV) light, also known as UV radiation. UV light is made up of several different types, or spectra, including UVA, UVB and UVC. (The different UV lights are distinguished by their wavelengths; UVA has the longest and UVC the shortest.) The atmosphere filters out all UVC light, so we don't have to worry about it. UVA light and UVB light cause most of the problems, and UVB appears to be the main culprit.

Here are some light facts:

- UVA outshines UVB 500-fold.

- UVB is more potent and penetrates more deeply.

- UVB is more responsible for sunburn and skin cancer than UVA.

- Even though 90 percent of UVB is sponged up by the outer layer of skin, it may still cause systemic (as well as skin) effects in people with lupus.

- UVA is responsible mainly for skin-related lupus reactions (for example, redness and discoid lesions).

- Infrared light—like the light from fire, which emits heat—can also cause a reaction, but it's much less common.

How Light Does Harm

You may remember that the lupus immune system seems mistakenly to target the body's own tissue as a foreign invader, not just harmful bacteria, viruses and other unwelcome visitors. Several things can go wrong when UV light shines on the lupus immune system: it can alter cells and make them more vulnerable to death or damage; it can directly kill cells; or it can alter the immune response. Here's how.

One common target of the immune system is the nuclei of cells. The nuclei hide so deeply inside the cells that they evade attack by the immune system's autoantibodies. But for some reason, the sun reacts profoundly with the skin cells of people who have lupus.

At lower exposure, the sun causes the nuclei to travel from their place deep inside the cells to the surfaces of the cells. The nuclei become exposed and accessible to autoantibodies, and the autoantibodies link up with the nuclei of the skin cells and kill them. Many experts believe this may be why UV light accentuates the skin lesions and facial rash seen in lupus patients.

At higher intensities, UV light directly kills skin cells; it doesn't need the help of autoantibodies. The cells fall apart and spill their contents—including DNA. Autoantibodies bind to DNA to form immune complexes. As you may remember, these immune complexes rove the blood system until they lodge somewhere—the kidney, the joints, the lungs—to cause inflammation. A flare results.

Finally, UV light can alter the immune system. One reason the sun causes skin cancer is that it calms down the immune system. This sounds like a good thing for people who have a hyperactive immune system—like people with lupus. But unfortunately, the UV light doesn't suppress autoantibodies. It suppresses other immune system activities, such as those that protect us against cancer. So people with lupus must be doubly warned about the sun: it not only triggers flares, but may make them more susceptible to skin cancer.

The Sun and Other UV Sources

Experts can't agree how much sun is okay and how much does harm. Some believe it's all right for even the most photosensitive to get a few minutes of sun a day—the risk of a sun reaction isn't enough to outweigh the benefits of getting a healthy dose of vitamin D. Other scientists argue that even the slightest hint of UV light should send photosensitive people running indoors, or at least to the store for protective clothing and sunscreen. Vitamin supplements can supply the vitamin D missing from sun exposure.

As with most aspects of lupus, your experience with the sun will be unique. Through cautious trial and error, you'll soon get a sense of how much UV light you can take.

Whether avoiding UV rays altogether or getting small doses, you should be aware of potential UV trouble spots. Not all are obvious. For example, if you think avoiding the sun on the hottest, clearest days will do the trick, think again. You can stroll through town on a cloudy day and still suffer a sun-related flare. The reason: clouds and fog are not dense enough to block UV rays; they're mainly made of water particles, and the rays just filter right through. UVA can reach you even through glass, so watch out when enjoying the view from a glassed-in porch, an airplane or even your car. Are you safe sitting in the shade? Not if your seat is near a body of water or other reflective surface, such as asphalt, plants or buildings.

Nor is the sun the only source of UVA and UVB light. The table below summarizes indoor origins. Generally speaking, the longer your level of exposure to the source of UV light, the greater your risk of a reaction. Some people may not react at all. Others are highly sensitive even to a short exposure. Some react to UVA light; others react to UVB light; still others react to both.

Table 6. Some Sources of UVA and UVB Light

	UVA	UVB
Sunlight (sunny or cloudy day)	X	X
Sunlight (through glass)	X	
Fluorescent light	X	X
X rays	X	
Photostatic copy machines	X	
Welding arcs	X	X
Tungsten iodide light (movie and slide projectors)	X	
Older color TV sets	X	

Photosensitizers

By virtue of having lupus, you're very likely to be photosensitized—that is, more sensitive to UV light. But a wide range of factors exist that may make you even more sensitive. A great many medications, for example, may heighten your sensitivity to the sun. Be sure to ask your doctor or pharmacist before taking even over-the-counter (nonprescription) drugs.

UV-light-sensitive people should also beware of eating

large amounts of foods containing psoralen, which may make them even more sensitive. These foods include celery, celery salt, parsnips, parsley and figs. It takes a lot of psoralen to cause sensitivity; to be safe, keep portions small.

Certain chemical and plant extracts may cause UV sensitivity. Ironically, certain agents in sunscreens such as PABA (see the list under "Evaluating Sunscreens"), benzophenones and cinnamates have been known to induce photosensitivity. Oil of citron, lavender, lime and other cosmetic preparations may also cause photosensitivity, including hexachlorophene in soaps, shampoos and deodorants. Hair dyes are implicated as well. For these reasons, many people with lupus use only "pure" products free of chemicals, dyes, and preservatives, such as those you'd buy in a "natural-products" store.

Finding Your Place in the Sun

Are you excluded from your place in the sun just because you have lupus? Certainly not—just take a few precautions:

- Wear sunscreen every day (see the list in the following section)—even when it's cloudy, even indoors. (Darker skin color may lessen your sensitivity to the sun in general, but black and Hispanic people with lupus are still vulnerable to a reaction.)

- Avoid direct exposure to the midday sun (between 10 a.m. and 4 p.m.). If you must go outside, wear sunscreen and protective clothing. Fabrics for hats and clothes should be of a tight weave (sheer fabrics let UV light through).

- Avoid tanning booths. Although they claim to emit safe UVA light, we know that UVA can cause problems.

- Make sure your sunglasses *and* regular eyeglasses are treated to absorb rays of UVA and UVB.

- Coat your car windows with special UV-absorbing films to allow safe daytime travel.

- Remember that UV light is intensified near water, snow and large open areas such as parking lots and fields.

- Keep in mind that your geographic location can influence the sun's intensity: UV light is more intense nearer the equator and at high altitudes (UV light is 20 percent more intense at 5,000 feet than at sea level).

Evaluating Sunscreens

Sunscreens work by bonding to the skin and absorbing the UV light before it gets to the skin. **Sunblocks** work by creating a physical barrier between the sun and the skin; zinc oxide, the white stuff lifeguards wear on their noses, is an example of a block. You may want to experiment with the colorful zinc oxides now available, but most people opt for sunscreens.

Growing scientific evidence of the sun's damaging effects has expanded the sunscreen market over the past few years. But not all sunscreens are alike. The most important variation is whether they protect against UVA and UVB or against just one wavelength.

Most sunscreens were designed to block UVB light. *The SPF, or Sun Protection Factor, applies only to UVB*

*protection. There is no standard for the UVA blocking
ability of a sunscreen.* Also, the SPF values in Europe
are different from those in the United States.

What does SPF really mean? The higher the SPF, the
longer the protection. If it normally takes you 10 minutes
in the sun to get a sunburn (or a photosensitivity reaction), an SPF of 15 will multiply that time by 15. In other
words, you should be able to tolerate the sun for 150 minutes instead of just 10. Most experts recommend a product with an SPF of at least 15, and some doctors say no
lower than SPF 25—the higher the better. The rule of
thumb is: the longer you want to stay outside, the higher
the SPF you should use.

But sunscreen wearer beware! Don't think that if you
continually reapply sunscreen you're extending your protection. Using SPF 15 extends your sun tolerance 15
times—period. Say it takes you 10 minutes to get a sun
reaction. An SPF 15 gives you 150 extra minutes—two
and a half more hours—in the sun. If you apply it at
noon, you're good until about 2:30 p.m. Suppose 2:30 rolls
around and you still want to stay out in the sun. Can you
extend your time another two and a half hours by re-
applying that SPF 15? No. You've used up your time in
the sun. Only if you go to a higher SPF will you be able
to stay out in the sun without a reaction.

The ingredients in sunscreens are important. Below we
list the ingredients in sunscreens and the spectrum of
light—UVA or UVB—they block. Of special note are
PABA and octyl p-dimethyl-aminobenzoate (which is
chemically related to PABA): both can cause skin reactions, a problem people with lupus certainly don't need.
In fact, if you're allergic to hair dyes, phenothiazine or
sulfonamide drugs, you may be sensitive to PABA.

Also of special interest is Parsol 1789 (a brand of
Givaudan Corporation), also known as avobenzone. This

new chemical provides the best UVA protection to date. Products are now available that combine the UVA protection of Parsol with the UVB protection of other chemicals.

While protection is important, staying power is also worth a look. A high-ranked SPF sunscreen can lose points if it can't stand up to heat, perspiration or water. Look for waterproof products: the oilier the product, the less likely it will be to wash off after contact with water. All products should be applied thirty minutes *before* going out into the sun and reapplied after swimming. Here are some chemical sunscreens and the UV screening they provide:

Para-aminobenzoic acid (PABA)—UVB
Cinnamates—UVB
Salicylates—UVB
Anthranilates—Some UVA and UVB
Parsol 1789—UVA
Benzophenones—UVA and some UVB

Medical Treatments

There are a number of ways to treat or prevent photosensitivity reactions. In brief, topical corticosteroids are usually used for skin lesions. If these don't work, dressings that keep steroids on the skin and injections may help.

If you find yourself needing repeated treatment for skin reactions by topical or injectable corticosteroids, you may be better suited for antimalarial therapy. Though somewhat controversial, antimalarials help extend your ability to tolerate the sun. See Chapter 5 for more about these drugs.

While your relationship with the sun may be particularly challenging, you're not alone. The entire world is looking at the sun with suspicion. It's hard to pick up a beauty or health magazine these days without reading something about the sun's harmful effects—especially as our earth's protective ozone layer shrinks. We've now learned that the term "healthy tan" is an oxymoron. Instead of being a sign of health, a tan betrays a risk of skin cancer and early skin aging. So if the risk of a flare doesn't inspire you to protect yourself, think of all those premature wrinkles!

A World of Allergens

It's amazing how often we continue to eat a certain food even when it makes us feel terrible. Usually we persevere because we don't make the connection between the food we love and a feeling we hate. Sometimes it just takes paying attention.

For people with lupus, paying attention can really pay off. We've read countless reports from patients about food sensitivities and other "allergies." Whether these reactions are true allergic responses or flares, many people with lupus have found that certain foods and substances (like wool or synthetic materials or hair dye) can aggravate symptoms. But sensitivity is a highly individual matter. You may have no problem with milk products, while someone else has a severe reaction. So it's up to you to be aware of substances that may send you into a flare.

Despite their individual nature, flares seem more common after exposure to certain substances. These include hydrazines (chemicals in some drugs, also found in some hair dyes, tobacco smoke and cooked, fatty foods), and asbestos and silica (silicone products found in breast implants).

Other substances seem to cause allergic reactions that mimic flares, including lactose (found in milk and other dairy products), which can cause cramping and stomach pain. Rashes and hives, common allergic reactions to foods, are also common symptoms of a lupus flare.

The bad news: flares are hard to distinguish from allergic reactions. The good news: it doesn't much matter. Either way, avoiding the offending substance averts the problem.

Colds, Flus and Flares

Though you don't catch lupus from a virus, it seems that viruses and bacteria can trigger a flare. We know that people with lupus get infections more often than other people. What we're not sure about—though it seems to be so from observation—is whether even a simple cold or flu can spur a lupus flare. Perhaps this results from the stresses put on the immune system when it is under attack by outside bacteria. Researchers do not yet know. In any case, there are *two* good reasons for you to get plenty of rest when you get a cold or flu: to get better more quickly and to limit the chance of a postinfection flare.

Stressing Your System

It hasn't been proved scientifically, but there are so many reports of stress-induced illnesses that a link is difficult to dismiss. New research shows that stress can change the immune system. The stress can be emotional (tension, anxiety or other emotional upset) or physical (injury, surgery or infection).

The idea, naturally, is to avoid stresses. Physical stresses may be difficult to avert: you often have little choice about surgery or accidents that cause physical harm. But you can try to control how far you stretch your physical resources. Overdoing it can send you into a flare, not to mention sapping your energy. Finding your balance between rest and activity is the key (see Chapter 8).

Emotional stresses are no less difficult to sidestep: they seem to come out of nowhere. It takes work to keep emotional calm in your life, especially with lupus. But it's important to try, since the consequences of upsets can set you back physically as well as emotionally. In Chapter 4 we looked at the sources of emotional stress in some depth and at ways you can help defuse them before they make you physically ill.

But let's face it, life is filled with stressors. If you can't avoid stress, at least be aware of it. After you've gone through an emotionally or physically stressful time, pay special attention to your body. It may be trying to warn you of an upcoming flare. If you respond, you may be able to avert or minimize a flare.

Medicines Can Trigger Lupus

There are a number of medications that can spur a lupus flare. If you want to avoid a flare, it makes sense to avoid these drugs. Agents such as estrogen-containing birth-control pills, hydralazine (used to treat high blood pressure), procainamide (heart drug), dilantin (used to treat epilepsy) and sulfonamides (antibiotics) can cause lupus flares. We included a more complete list of these agents in Chapter 1.

Signals of a Flare

Even after you've been diagnosed and are taking medications to control your symptoms, you may still be vulnerable to a flare. When your body goes into a flare phase, it sends out alarms. Tuning in to your body's warnings can spare you a lot of time out of commission because the earlier you treat a flare, the better it can be controlled.

Lupus is a disease that repeats itself. With experience, you'll come to know the symptoms of an upcoming flare. And since each person's experience with lupus is unique, your symptoms will probably be different from someone else's. Take note of the early signs. When you start having "that certain feeling," don't hesitate to call your doctor. He or she will try to help you preempt the full-blown effects.

Lupus may also evolve. After years of experiencing one pattern, you may suddenly acquire a new symptom.

Here are a few of the most common warning signs of a flare:

- **You get tired more easily or more often.** This is a clear signal from your body to stop or slow down and get some help from your physician.

- **You feel more pain.** If pain commonly is part of your flare, don't ignore increasing pain. It could mount to a full-blown flare.

- **A rash grows.** Like increasing pain, a growing rash could be the start of a flare. Take heed and get the right treatment.

- **You have a fever of 100 degrees Fahrenheit or more for three or more days.** This is a common signal of an immune reaction and inflammation.

- **Your stomach hurts.** Often the digestive system goes out of whack when the body is getting ready to inflame.

- **You have trouble breathing.** Here is another sign that your immune system is getting out of order.

- **You have a headache, dizziness and blurred vision.** All may presage a flare.

- **Your urine is red or cloudy.** This may foreshadow a kidney-related flare.

Again, your symptoms are unique. Should you feel familiar hints, do your best to stop your symptoms from progressing by speaking with your physician. It could make the difference between a mild flare (or none at all) and a long-lasting one.

Seven Steps to Preventing a Flare

To sum up this chapter, here are some practical steps you can take to sidestep a flare:

1. Find your place in the sun. Are you among the 60 percent of people with lupus who are sensitive to UV light? Can you sustain small amounts or large amounts? Learn your limits; then keep within them.

2. Know and avoid UV light sources. The sun isn't the only culprit: fluorescent lights are also common sources of UV rays.

3. Avoid photosensitizers. Know which medications, chemicals and foods aggravate UV-sensitivity.

4. Practice UV light control. Using sunscreens (PABA-free) and wearing protective clothing should be daily practices.

5. Keep tabs on emotional ups and downs. Recognize that an emotional upset can trigger a flare. If you've just gone through an emotional time, pay closer attention to your body for early warnings of a flare.

6. Avoid flare-triggering medications. See Chapter 1 for an inclusive list of medications that may initiate a flare.

7. Tune in to your body's warning signs. Know those first signals of a flare and get early treatment; the earlier you get help, the better your chances of controlling the flare.

CHAPTER 7

Pregnancy and Parenthood

If you have lupus and you're considering pregnancy, you probably have many questions: Can I get pregnant? What are the risks to me and my child? Is it safe to continue with my medications? Will I pass lupus on to my baby? Can I cope with a newborn and toddler?

Having discoid lupus only carries no additional risk in pregnancy, compared to the general population. The issue is less clear-cut for women with systemic disease. There was a time when mothers with lupus rarely survived pregnancy, and it was all but prohibited. Today, while flares can occur during and after pregnancy, it's often hard to know the relationship between pregnancy and flares. What we can say is that *for most women, systemic lupus has no effect on fertility or pregnancy, and pregnancy has no effect on the disease.*

There's probably more fear than real threat attached to lupus and pregnancy. While risks exist for women with lupus, proper planning and close monitoring can be powerful allies in achieving a healthy pregnancy.

The question whether you can cope with parenthood is

one you should consider carefully—with your mate and with your physician, if you wish—before trying to conceive. Having a child, as you doubtless know, requires physical and emotional energy. Talking with other mothers who have lupus, and mothers who don't, might be one way to prepare for the joys and challenges ahead.

In this chapter, we'll address the issues of concern to women with lupus who wish to become pregnant, with the caveat that your individual condition is the most important determinant of your fertility and your reaction to pregnancy. We'll also look at the challenges facing parents of children with lupus.

Having a Baby

Even though 50 percent of all lupus pregnancies are completely normal, they all should be considered high-risk. Extra care should be taken to monitor the progress of the woman and the fetus throughout the pregnancy. "High-risk" is a scary term. Really, it just signifies conservative measures—a "better safe than sorry" approach. Women with lupus should work with a doctor familiar with high-risk pregnancies (ideally, your obstetrician or midwife will be in contact with your lupus caregiver, whether that caregiver is a rheumatologist or a primary care physician), and should plan to deliver at a hospital equipped to handle premature newborns.

Severe Disease Poses More Problems in Pregnancy

The good news is that pregnancy rates among women with lupus are close to those of the general population: about 80 percent can conceive, compared to 90 percent in the general population. But some women with lupus, mostly those with severe disease, may have specific problems.

One of the greatest concerns among women with severe lupus is irregular periods and whether they affect the ability to conceive. Amenorrhea, or lack of menstruation, may temporarily turn off your fertility—or you may still ovulate even if you don't have a period. Figuring out which are your fertile days may be a challenge, though, and may call for the aid of the ovulation predictor tests now available.

Spontaneous abortion is also a considerable problem among women with severe lupus. In addition, women with uremia are less likely to conceive. (Uremia is a condition often related to nephritis whereby waste products normally filtered out of the blood are retained.)

Should women with severe lupus give up on pregnancy? Not without a thorough look at all the options. It may be more difficult for you to become pregnant or to carry the child to term, but each person is unique. Have a talk with your doctor about the strategies that are right for you.

Certain medications can definitely get in the way of fertility. Long-term treatment with cyclophosphamide can affect the function of the ovaries, causing irregular menstrual periods and infertility. Fertility sometimes returns after stopping the drug, but infertility may be permanent. (See the following sections for more about medications during pregnancy.)

Pregnancy and Flares

Is it pregnancy, or is it a flare? Lupus, the "great imitator," mimics pregnancy as well. Many symptoms of pregnancy are easily mistaken for early signals of a flare: fluid in the joints may cause swelling similar to that of arthritis; higher blood flow can cause a redness in the face that may look like a lupus rash; hair loss may seem like a flare warning, but actually it's a normal occurrence in pregnant women.

Some experts believe that pregnancy awakens symptoms in 25 percent of women with lupus. Others assert that pregnancy is just as likely to send a woman with lupus into a flare as into remission. Unless you have severe kidney or cardiac disease, you may have flares, but being pregnant won't make them worse.

The Kidney, the Heart and Pregnancy

Women with kidney involvement are at higher risk than others with lupus. Up to 50 percent will have a flare if they get pregnant while their disease is active.

Certain conditions prohibit pregnancy: a high serum creatinine level, greater than 2 mg/dl (milligrams per deciliter), indicating impaired kidney function; severe high blood pressure and a condition known as nephrotic syndrome, which means having higher than normal amounts of protein in the urine. Women with these conditions who get pregnant put themselves at considerable risk.

Women with severe heart involvement are also at greater risk for complications with the fetus, or harm to themselves, during pregnancy. If you have such involvement, speak with your physician about your condition.

Timing Your Pregnancy

The best time to get pregnant is when you feel your best. Most doctors agree that, if you can, you should time your pregnancy during a period of remission. Becoming pregnant during an active phase of lupus puts a lot of stress on your body. Imagine morning sickness during a flare!

Stories about pregnancy's ability to "solve" a flare are untrue. So if your disease is active, try to resolve symptoms before you conceive.

Keep a Close Watch

Even women who conceive during remission face potential risks throughout pregnancy. One-third of women have antiphospholipid antibodies, which put them at higher risk for early miscarriage; and one-fifth have preeclampsia/toxemia, a dangerous condition that necessitates early delivery.

Antiphospholipid antibodies are a family of antibodies that include anticardiolipin, antiphosphatidylserine, and lupus anticoagulant. If you test positive for any of these components, or if you have a false positive result for syphilis, you may be at higher risk for fetal loss, which often happens midpregnancy. If it strikes late enough in the pregnancy, the baby may be delivered normally, although prematurely. Treatment to prevent fetal loss is controversial. Corticosteroids, aspirin and plasmapheresis are being tested. And even though one-third of women with lupus have antiphospholipid antibodies, many still have normal pregnancies.

Preeclampsia, or toxemia of pregnancy, is very serious. Symptoms include climbing high blood pressure, headaches, protein in the urine and swelling of the lower extremities. If it isn't treated right away, preeclampsia can lead to coma or death. This problem is most common among women who are older, black, have kidney disease, have high blood pressure, smoke or are carrying twins. Often preeclampsia requires immediate delivery of the baby. If the condition is caught early enough, though, there should be no danger to the mother. Signs of preeclampsia include the symptoms mentioned above, as well as abnormal serum complement and platelet counts.

Medications During Pregnancy

You've probably read that all medicines should be avoided during pregnancy. Like tobacco and alcohol, medicines can negatively influence the formation of the fetus. All lupus drugs *may* affect the baby's formation—some very rarely, some very commonly. It's imperative to weigh the benefits of treatment and the risks of side effects to you and your baby. You always take some degree of risk when you use medications during pregnancy. But you may also risk a lupus flare and your own health if you stop taking them. The decision isn't easy.

Antimalarials taken by the mother may accumulate in the eyes of newborns. But this is very rare, and most studies of pregnant mothers and their children fail to prove any harm caused by antimalarials taken during pregnancy.

Aspirin and other nonsteroidal antiinflammatory drugs (NSAIDs) can bring circulation-related problems. Just as they thin the blood of adults who take them, NSAIDs can cause bleeding and circulation problems among both mothers and newborns.

Corticosteroids are often continued during pregnancy, with only rare ill effects on the mother or the fetus (or newborn). These effects include cleft palate, masculinizaton of female infants, adrenal insufficiency, low birth weight and dependency on corticosteroids.

Most **cytotoxic drugs** are strictly prohibited during pregnancy. Cyclophosphamide and chlorambucil are known to cause defects and abortion. Some evidence suggests that azathioprine may be a safer alternative, but the jury is still out.

Lupus and the Newborn

Only 2 percent of children inherit lupus from their parents. However, the incidence of rheumatic diseases (immune diseases that affect connective tissue) is higher among offspring of people with lupus.

Birth defects are rare, in spite of the use of medications during pregnancy.

About 25 to 30 percent of people with lupus have an antibody called anti-Ro or anti-SSA. Ten percent of these women deliver babies with neonatal lupus (lupus that afflicts only newborns). Sometimes women who have the anti-Ro antibody show no symptoms—the delivery of a child with neonatal lupus is the first sign that the mother has lupus.

If you remember the discussion from Chapter 1, neonatal lupus is a syndrome very different from other types of lupus. First, it affects only newborns. Most signs disappear without a trace after six months. Second, most symptoms are very mild and nonthreatening, including rashes and unimportant blood count abnormalities. But a very few children of lupus mothers, 3 percent, will also have heart block, a condition that does not disappear.

Most children develop normally in spite of it; a few require pacemakers, and a very few do not survive.

There are treatments for the symptoms of neonatal lupus; they include medications and keeping the baby out of the sun.

Breast-feeding

The decision whether or not to breast-feed is partly medical and partly personal. In and of itself, breast-feeding is not harmful to the mother with lupus, though it may be tiring for her. But for the mother taking medications, breast-feeding may bring some harm to the child. Though very little is known about how lupus medicines affect breast-fed infants, some drugs may be passed on through breast milk.

If you want to err on the conservative side, you probably should avoid all medications during breast-feeding, including over-the-counter medicines, nicotine and alcohol. Choose either breast-feeding or medication—not both.

But if you want to decide based on scanty medical proof, you'll find some reports that low doses of prednisone (less than 30 milligrams per day) produce no problems. While one camp of experts say that aspirin and NSAIDs are okay, others believe high doses may affect the child's blood system. Women taking cyclophosphamides should definitely not breast-feed their infants.

Should You Test Your Baby for Lupus?

If you see signs of neonatal lupus, your baby needs medical attention and should be tested for neonatal lupus. But for the majority of babies, testing is not recommended.

First of all, a lupus diagnosis is based on much more than a laboratory test. As we discussed in Chapter 2, there is no test for lupus. Diagnosis is made only after a patient has met the eleven criteria.

Second, even if your baby has tested positive for antibodies (ANA or anti-Sm, for example), that doesn't mean she or he has lupus. Antibodies easily cross the placenta and show up in the infant's blood—the mother, not the baby, is producing them. As the baby starts making her or his own antibodies, this picture may change. So tests can be misleading in the early days of an infant's life.

Lupus in the Family

In Chapter 4, we covered many of the challenges facing a parent who has lupus. But what about the parent of a child who has lupus?

When a child has lupus, it's a family condition. It's common for parents to feel responsible for their children's plight. Guilt, anger, fear, blame—the host of emotions that tag along with the disease—invade the hearts of many parents whose children have lupus. Parents face a double challenge: coping with their own emotions and caring for their child. Both require attention, patience and clearheadedness.

Parents, know that you're not alone. Your physicians (we'll discuss this later), and possibly a family counselor, can help you sort out practical steps toward the mental and physical health of your family. In the pages that follow, we'll help you get started.

Childhood Symptoms

About 20 percent of people with lupus first have symptoms as a child, as early as the age of three. The first symptoms of lupus are the same as they are for adults, but with more fever and arthritis.

Just like lupus in adults, lupus in children is hard to diagnose. Symptoms creep up slowly and are easy to confuse with those of other conditions. Symptoms like fever and fatigue are hard to separate from the normal illnesses of children. Children are more prone to fever than adults. The eleven criteria for diagnosing lupus, outlined in Chapter 2, hold true for children.

Parents who have lupus carry a greater burden. Because of their own experience, they may be especially watchful and overanxious about small signs of lupus-like symptoms. It's important to avoid jumping to conclusions based on a fever or aches and pains. But if these symptoms continue for no reason, a lupus workup may be in order.

Your Child's Health Care Team

Children with lupus often need extra medical care. Few pediatricians have the expertise to treat the complex symptoms and immune problems that come up with lupus. A pediatrician is still needed to help manage normal childhood conditions and vaccinations. But a pediatric rheumatologist, a doctor who specializes in immune-related disorders of children, should also be consulted.

Not all towns have rheumatologists, much less pediatric rheumatologists. You may need a recommendation from your local doctor, or to call your state's medical association, or to contact the American College of Rheumatology (address in the "Resources" section at the end of this book).

Ideally, your regular pediatrician and your pediatric rheumatologist will work together in the best interest of your child. You may need to help coordinate communication between the pediatrician and rheumatologist. Your pediatrician should be aware of your child's lupus and treatment guidelines. (For example, most vaccines seem to work just as well in people with lupus as they do in other people, but some, such as tetanus, may be slightly less effective (especially when given during corticosteroid therapy).

Your child's school administration—principal, medical staff and teachers—should be aware of the symptoms of lupus. While children with lupus shouldn't get special treatment, they may need more rest than other children. Understanding some of the special needs of children with lupus allows school staff members to make the necessary allowances.

Do's and Don't's for Parents

It's often easy to forget that there's a child behind the lupus—a child who needs the love (not the pity) of her or his parents, who needs freedom to grow and learn. Here are some tips to help you keep a balance between proper care and overprotectiveness:

- **Do learn about lupus.** Become a lupus expert. You may have rushed straight to this section. Know that childhood lupus is similar to that of adults. The information in this book applies to children, too.

- **Don't pity your child.** There are few things more painful to parents than seeing their children ill. It's tempting to overindulge such children—especially when nothing else seems to make them feel better. While it's true that your child needs some special care—and some understanding—she or he should be encouraged to behave like other children. Your attitude can mean the difference between making your child feel "less than" and helping her or him to feel "normal." The child with lupus should be subject to the same house rules as the other children—within reason. She or he may need more rest than the others and may not bear up well under strenuous household tasks. Instead of assigning this child lawn work, give her or him kitchen duty.

- **Do encourage self-awareness.** It's not easy for children to understand why they can't do what other kids do. Your child might fight treatment, question it or try to deny that her or his lupus exists. With the help of your physician, give the child the information needed to understand any restrictions. You may get tired of continually explaining the need to take medication, to avoid the sun or wear sunscreen and to rest, but explanations help to educate your child.

- **Don't forget your other kids.** This sounds obvious, but siblings may feel left out when they see the child with lupus getting all the attention. Lupus is a family affair, but for brothers and sisters who don't really understand lupus (and how can they be expected to?), it's just a drag. They may need to be educated and to be reminded how important they are—even though they're healthy.

- **Do conquer guilt.** Know that lupus is not inherited. It cannot be caught, like a flu or a cold. It does not come from the food you eat. In short, *there's nothing you could have done to keep your child from getting lupus.* So don't be guilty; be a parent. If you feel unhappy and guilty, your child will feel the same way. Take the action needed to deal with the situation as it exists today.

- **Don't ignore your own needs.** Caring for your child and your family is rewarding, but it can also be draining. Take time out for yourself and your spouse. It may be difficult, but find some time to do things you *enjoy.*

CHAPTER 8

Lifestyle Lessons

The quality of your life with lupus depends on many factors: the severity of your disease, your attitude toward illness and how well you take care of yourself. We've already looked at the ways lupus can affect the body and the ways your emotional outlook can affect your health. We've also touched on some of the lifestyle guidelines that can help prevent or avert a flare. But what about the basics of your daily life—the foods you eat, the kind and amount of activity you engage in, your personal care?

We look forward to great advances in therapeutic nutrition—scientists are beginning to test nutritional claims for plants and foods using rigorous modern research methods. But until studies are conducted and we read convincing evidence that special diets or vitamins are at least as good as today's medicines, we can't in good conscience recommend nutritional approaches to living with lupus.

However, there's no doubt that a well-balanced diet is vital to good health. And following certain diet and exercise guidelines can make living with lupus a little easier. But please don't read this chapter expecting dietary or exercise "remedies." Rather, you'll find proven lifestyle tips to help you cope with symptoms and drug side effects.

Furthermore, people with lupus often struggle to keep a balance between fatigue and energy. Rest figures prominently on our agenda of daily "activities." How can you get the most out of the energy you have? What about exercise? This chapter will explore these issues as well.

Finally, we'll look at personal care, such as cosmetics and soaps. People with discoid lupus, or systemic lupus with skin involvement, are often in a quandary about the best types of products to use. The suggestions at the end of this chapter should help.

Some Diet Do's and Don't's

The foods on the following list of dietary offenders and helpers are probably familiar to you. They're the same ones you see every day in articles about health. But for people with lupus, eating or avoiding these foods has more than general dietary health significance.

- **Don't drink caffeine.** Caffeine—found in coffee, tea and many soda pops—is a powerful stimulant. Stimulants can raise the heart rate and add to stress. Stress can trigger flares. Get the connection? Caffeine can also cause stomach problems, which you don't need if you're already taking NSAIDs for flare relief.

  Quitting caffeine is not easy. Quitters often fail because they try to do it suddenly. Abrupt withdrawal from caffeine can cause severe symptoms— headaches and irritability are among the more common. That's why experts recommend taking a week to taper off. For the first three days, get your caffeine down to one cup a day. For the next two days, drink half decaffeinated and half caffeinated coffee. For the next two days, drink one-quarter caffeinated and three-quarters decaffeinated coffee. By the next week, you should be able to drink decaffeinated coffee or tea without symptoms.

- **Do limit fat and cholesterol.** Fat and cholesterol are especially bad for people taking corticosteroids. As you probably know, high cholesterol levels (caused by foods that are high in saturated fat and cholesterol) are connected with heart disease. Since corticosteroids also have the same effect, you could be doubling your risk.

  Look for foods that are low in saturated fat. According to the U.S. Surgeon General, fat should make up 30 percent or less of your daily caloric intake. How fat-laden is your diet? Food labels will soon make it easy to figure out by displaying the fat content as a percentage of total calories. But until that happens, here's how to calculate it yourself: First, figure out how many calories a food has per serving. Suppose the food is a "low-fat" frozen yogurt dessert, with 150 calories per serving. Next, scan the label for the grams of fat per serving, which we'll say is 6. Now, how do you know whether this is less or more than 30 percent of the calories? There are 9 calories per gram of fat. So multiply the grams of fat per serving by 9. Then divide by the total calories per serving:

$$\textbf{(Grams of fat} \times \textbf{9)} \div \textbf{(total calories)} = \textbf{\% fat}$$
$$\textbf{per serving}$$

Using our example, we have *54 (6 grams of fat multiplied by 9 calories per gram).* When we divide 54 by 150 (total calories), we get .36; the percent of fat per serving, then, is 36. So according to our new fat math, the "low-fat" frozen yogurt dessert just skims past the recommended allowance. Not so low-fat after all.

Not all fat is created equal. The kind of fat that raises cholesterol levels is called saturated fat. Butter, for example, is high in saturated fat. Many vegetable oils, such as olive oil and canola oil, are high in fat, but the fat is unsaturated. So it's better to cook with canola or olive oil than butter.

Unfortunately, many foods don't include labels. How do you tell okay (unsaturated) fats from bad (saturated) fats? Fats that are liquid or semiliquid at room temperature are unsaturated fats. Fats that are solid in a cool kitchen, such as meat fat and sausage, butter and lard, are saturated fats. Dairy foods are also high in fat. Eggs and shellfish are not high in saturated fat, but they are high in cholesterol.

Do you have to give up all dairy foods? Absolutely not. In fact, these foods can be important sources of vitamin D and calcium. So opt instead for the growing number of low-fat or no-fat versions of milk, yogurt, cream cheese and even mayonnaise.

- **Do include foods high in fiber.** While they are not common primary problems among people with lupus, many of us suffer gastric upset, heartburn and bloating as the result of many factors. A high-fiber diet can help keep us regular and keep the colon healthy. Foods that are high in fiber include fresh fruits and vegetables, whole-grain bread, brown rice, peas and beans.

- **Do limit salt intake.** As with fat, a high-salt diet is a known contributor to heart disease, so it should be avoided in people taking corticosteroids, which can raise blood pressure and cause arteriosclerosis with long-term use. Also, if you have kidney involvement, especially if you have high blood pressure and fluid retention, it's extremely important to avoid salt.

  Americans are chronic oversalters, and a salt-free diet may seem bland. To add variety to your culinary life, use spices. Or simply learn to enjoy the tastes of all the fresh fruits and vegetables you're now eating because you're also lowering your fat intake.

- **Don't expect too much from vitamin supplements.** A well-balanced diet that meets the daily requirements for vitamins and minerals is essential to everyone's health—but especially to the health of people with lupus.

  With a few exceptions, there's little evidence that vitamin supplements—except in the case of documented deficiency—are of any real value in making symptoms easier to handle. It's much better for your body to get as many vitamins as possible from foods. If you plan your diet to provide a wide range of vitamins and minerals, you'll have less room for "empty" calories, so you'll probably see a positive improvement in your weight as well.

  People with photosensitivity who avoid the sun may lack vitamin D. But taking vitamin D supplements is controversial. There's some evidence that vitamin deficiencies can trigger flares. Whether this requires a vitamin supplement depends on the foods you eat and other basic health criteria that are unique to you. It's important to discuss these issues with your physician, since high doses of vitamins can cause serious health problems.

- **Do get plenty of minerals.** People with lupus-related anemia may benefit from iron supplements. Those taking prednisone for long periods, or at high doses, are subject to osteoporosis, or bone thinning. Calcium has proved valuable in combating osteoporosis. Again, consult your physician for the right formulations and doses of these supplements.

Balance Rest and Activity

No one can tell better than you when you're ready to drop from exhaustion. Wholesale advice like "rest three hours a day" simply does not meet the highly individual needs of people with lupus. Some people require more rest; others do fine with less. In fact, your rest:activity quotient probably changes from month to month, depending on how active your disease is. Indeed, finding the right amount of rest for you is a balancing act.

Here are some principles to help you find that balance.

- **The more active the disease, the less active you should be.** You probably won't have much of a choice. Accepting that your body needs to rest—*insists* on rest—is one of the major challenges of having lupus. Try not to judge the desire to rest. Your mind might be awhirl with lists of tasks and goals, with guilt and anger, but try to take it easy. Listen to your body, not your mind. Your body will thank you by recovering faster.

- **Avoid overcompensating.** At last you feel better. Now you can get to all the things you put off while you were sick, right? Wrong. It's a natural impulse to want to overdo it while feeling good, to make up for lost time. But there's no better way to send yourself right back into a flare. Try to find a happy medium. (See "Setting the Pace" on page 168.) You deserve to enjoy your healthy time.

- **Get exercise, but set limits.** Unless your condition absolutely prohibits it, exercise is a positive activity. Contrary to outdated beliefs, exercise is just as healthy for people with lupus as it is for the general population. But again, exercise has its limits—and it's up to you to set them.

  If you sense a flare coming on—a flu-like feeling—maybe it's best to go easy on the exercise. Also, don't exercise to the point of utter exhaustion; this could injure your body and stress your system to the brink of a flare. On the other hand, if you're in the middle of a remission, there's no reason to avoid exercise. The basic tenets of exercise hold true for everyone, including people with lupus: build your exercise tolerance slowly.

  For some people with lupus, exercise is actually therapeutic. People with myositis, or muscle inflammation, may be subject to a wasting away of muscle. People with lupus arthritis may have limited range of motion. Those of you taking corticosteroids may be at risk of osteoporosis. Regular, supervised exercise can help build muscle mass, keep joints mobile and strengthen bones. See "Exercise Tips" on page 170.

Setting the Pace

How do you put the principles outlined above into practice? Here are some pointers:

- **Set priorities.** You can't do everything during a remission, and you can do even less during a flare. What's the solution to this frustrating state of affairs? Priorities. If you're not naturally inclined to organize your time and plan your day, make a list. What would you like to accomplish during the period you have? After reviewing this wish list, prioritize it. What is a must-do? A can-do-without?

  Take one activity at a time, starting with your number-one must-do. Once that task is accomplished, take a break and listen to your body. Are you tired? Don't ignore the signs of an upcoming flare (see Chapter 6) or you may pay for it tomorrow, and possibly for days after that.

  If you feel fine, continue with your list. Remember, if you accomplish just one thing on a low-energy day, you've done a lot. It's much better to do one thing and have energy to spare than to do three things that leave you exhausted at the end of the day. By reserving your energy for the most important goals, you preserve more energy to accomplish more the next day.

- **Rearrange the furniture?** When you have lupus, every calorie of energy can be precious. During times of disease activity, it may be wise to examine your regular patterns for energy-draining movements. You'll be surprised how much energy you waste without even knowing it. The changes you make may be major, like spreading your chores throughout the week rather than accomplishing them all at once, or minor, like buying rollers for your furniture to make moving it easier.

Robert Phillips, author of *Coping with Lupus*, offers some excellent suggestions, such as wearing clothes that are easier to get in and out of, lubricating drawers so that they glide more smoothly and installing larger drawer pulls.

Other suggestions: Install an answering machine to catch calls, rather than run for the phone. Reorganize your closet or kitchen so that often-used objects are easier to reach and put away. Invest a few dollars in some work-saving household devices, like a squeegee for cleaning mirrors and windows.

- **Schedule rest periods.** You're in the middle of a busy day and you feel great. But it's still important to take some time to rest. Schedule frequent, short rest stops in the middle of your day and you'll be able to sustain your energy longer.

- **Get outside help.** It's not easy to let go of activities. Some people feel as if it's admitting failure or giving in to the disease. Others may feel a loss of self-worth, since our identities are often so wrapped up with our actions and accomplishments.

And it's one thing to cut an activity from your schedule; it's another thing to hand the responsibility over to someone else. You may feel like a burden to others, that you're not indispensable, that you're of little value to your family and friends.

Realize that your life is at stake: you're worth very little to yourself or anyone else after you work yourself to the point of a bone-tiring flare. Also, you're not the only one who feels helpless in the face of your lupus. If those who love you can't make you well, they can at least make your life easier. Your teenagers might not get your laundry as white as you like it, but practice makes perfect. Your neighbor probably won't mind bringing you a few things from the grocery store every so often. Your friends would probably love to do something for you, like pick up your dry cleaning.

Give your loved ones a chance to give to you. It's only natural.

Exercise Tips

- Consult your physician before starting any exercise program. This is good advice for anyone, but especially useful for people with lupus, who may benefit from specific pointers from their physicians.

- Exercise moderately to relieve tension and build strength. You don't have to work yourself into an aerobic sweat to benefit from exercise.

- Build your exercise time and train slowly. Rather than stress your body and your system by overdoing it, go slow. You'll be surprised at how effective slow and steady exercise can be.

- Know the signs of too much exercise. Exhaustion, muscle and joint stiffness, and pain are signals that you should slow down.

- Know which exercises are best for your condition. See Table 7 on page 171 for the right type of exercise to help build endurance, muscle strength, bone strength or joint strength.

**Table 7. Recommended Exercises for
People with Lupus**

Condition	Aim of Exercise	Suitable Exercise
Lupus myositis (inflammation of muscle)	Build muscle strength	Swimming, walking, isometrics
Corticosteroid-induced osteoporosis	Build bone strength	Weight-bearing exercises (walking, aerobics, step aerobics)
Lupus arthritis	Free range of motion (avoid joint stress)	Stretching, swimming, yoga, isometrics
Lupus fatigue	Endurance	Gentle aerobic exercise (swimming, walking)

Beauty and the Wolf

We've talked a little about the emotional problems that arise when lupus strikes the skin. But what about some practical, day-to-day advice for the care of sensitive lupus skin?

Few doctors concern themselves with the issue of beauty. But patients certainly do. And through trial and error, patients have arrived at some very sensible skin maintenance regimens that we would recommend to anyone.

Here are some tried-and-true tips from Jill Elias, who has struggled with discoid lupus for more than ten years.

This regimen, based on using all-natural, plant-based products, has helped Elias significantly reduce flares on her very sensitive skin.

- Cleanse your face thoroughly twice a day using noncomedogenic, hypoallergenic, perfume-free, 100 percent natural products.

- Avoid using alcohol-based products regularly; they may irritate the skin. Try witch hazel instead.

- Use oatmeal as a gentle facial wash; use oatmeal baths to soothe and cleanse the skin. Or try perfume-, alcohol- and chemical-free mineral baths such as a clay cleanser.

- Avoid soaps and other surface-acting chemicals, which can also harm the skin.

- Rather than rub skin dry with a towel, allow it to air-dry.

- Apply a nongreasy moisturizer to moist skin after a bath and allow to air-dry.

- Moisturize your face with a light, hypoallergenic, noncomedogenic product. For daytime use, try one with SPF.

- In cities, wear a light foundation (many are available with SPF) under makeup for pollution protection during the day.

- Avoid chemical hair dyes; opt for natural henna colors instead. The hydrazines in many hair dyes may trigger a flare.

- Since the alcohol in perfume can irritate the skin, spray it on clothing and hair instead.

- It may be tempting to scratch or rub your face, but try not to touch or fuss with it too much.

CHAPTER 9

New Horizons

This book is filled with facts, but it leaves two important questions unanswered: what causes lupus and what will cure it? Though we've come to the end of the book, lupus research continues. Scientists are now exploring the mysterious origins of the disease. They're working on more effective and gentler ways of treating it. And as we learn more about lupus, a cure does not seem so distant.

Here are some of the advances now being investigated—advances that will help people with lupus today, and in generations to come.

More Learning About Lupus

Though we do not know what causes lupus, researchers have some ideas, based on physiological, and just plain logical, clues.

For example, researchers have long suspected that a virus may somehow play a role in lupus. Though it's clear that a virus alone can't cause lupus (otherwise more than just 500,000 people would have it), it may represent a piece of the puzzle.

Pursuit of a retrovirus has uncovered some fascinating leads. A retrovirus is a virus that infiltrates the body and becomes part of its genes, then goes into a dormant state. Since the body can't eliminate an inactive virus, the dormant virus is free to act slowly (chronically) or sporadically (acutely)—much the way lupus expresses itself. Another clue to a potential retrovirus involvement is the fact that certain autoantibodies in some people with lupus and with Sjogren's syndrome (a related immune disorder) bind to one particular retrovirus. The discovery of a retrovirus related to immune disorders is an exciting one, but much more research is needed before any conclusions can be reached.

Though lupus is not inherited, there is a greater tendency for family members to have immune disorders. So perhaps part of the problem is in our genes. This theory is being borne out by animal research. Some researchers have found that a certain gene has been linked with fewer or less severe symptoms in lupus-afflicted mice. The new gene seems to turn off the production of B cells that make antibodies against DNA. But it leaves alone the B cells that make other necessary antibodies. Scientists pursue genetic research with the hope that it may lead to therapy for humans.

Other genetic research attempts to discover why healthy family members of people with lupus sometimes carry the anti-DNA antibody. Some scientists think there may be a factor that makes a person more prone to developing lupus.

The autoantibodies made only by people with lupus—anti-DNA and anti-Sm—inspire other lupus researchers. They've found that some antibodies react against more than one antigen. This might mean that autoantibodies against DNA might very well be produced in response to something besides DNA, perhaps something from the environment. The disease process could be triggered by some outside force, then picked up and perpetuated by the body's DNA.

Following the trail of immune complexes—those substances that cause inflammation and tissue damage—leads to some interesting theories. We know that people with lupus have more immune complexes than other people. Is this because the body produces more, or because it can't get rid of them fast enough? It appears that the latter may be true (which doesn't mean the former can't be true, too). The body usually rids itself of immune complexes with the help of complement. But if complement lacks a receptor for the immune complex—meaning it can't recognize the immune complex or grab hold of it—the immune complex will build up in the system with nothing to escort it out. This may be the case in people with lupus, who seem to have a receptor defect. This defect may be inherited, or it may be acquired.

Since women of childbearing age are at highest risk of systemic lupus, scientists are intrigued by the role of estrogen in lupus. In animal studies, higher levels of female hormones tend to accelerate lupus, while male hormones like testosterone tend to suppress it. To do their job in regulating female function, estrogens seem either to increase anti-DNA or to lower the ability of the body to get rid of immune complexes. Some researchers have found that males and females with lupus have a hard time using estrogen—and levels of testosterone are lower than normal in women with lupus. Also, levels of male hormones were much lower in women with active disease than in either normal women or women with inactive disease.

One scientist believes that lupus is not caused by a misguided immune system but by defects in the lupus DNA which the immune system perceives as threatening. As a result, the immune system launches an attack against the body's own genetic factory.

These are just a few of the more promising concepts being explored—some of which may one day lead to a cure for lupus.

Changes in Treatment

While some researchers follow clues to a cure, others focus on the problems of today: making existing treatments as effective as possible, or creating new treatments.

Much new research centers on the more severe expressions of lupus, such as nephritis and vasculitis. When a kidney is damaged beyond repair or treatment, a kidney transplant may be in order. The challenge has been to get the lupus immune system to accept the foreign kidney. Highly toxic drugs have often been given to calm down the immune system. New drugs that are less toxic and more effective now make kidney transplants almost as easy for people with lupus to accept as others.

Under normal conditions, the body tolerates all the different parts of itself. In lupus, the immune system perceives certain parts of its own body as foreign invaders, and mounts an attack. Research is under way to **induce tolerance of self antigens;** that is, to help the body learn to accept itself. This is done by linking the rejected substance with an accepted substance. For example, suppose the body rejects DNA as foreign and threatening. If DNA can be attached to an acceptable substance, like the antibody IgG, the body may be more disposed toward accepting it. This approach may sound like science fiction, but it's actually working in animal studies.

Plasmapheresis is a process by which the plasma of people with severe disease is withdrawn and replaced with fresh plasma. In **plasma exchange,** plasma is withdrawn so that the immune complexes can be filtered out, and oxygen-carrying red cells are put back in their place. This procedure is also becoming more widely used.

Extracorporeal immunoadsorption is a procedure by which disease-causing antibodies and immune complexes are removed from the blood by hemodialysis (through filtering tubes). The tubes are bathed in substances that attract and remove (adsorb) the immune complexes and return the healthy parts of the blood to the circulation.

Total nodal irradiation is a procedure that calms the immune system. It's a form of very specific radiation therapy. It has the advantage of targeting the lymph organs, the immune system's "control center." While it's not without side effects, total nodal irradiation is less toxic than cyclophosphamides and other cytotoxic drugs, which also suppress immune activity.

Ancrod is a new drug used to help people who have severe disease, including very small blood clots. Still in the early stages of development, this drug may be helpful for people with thrombosis of the eye, retina and deep veins, or with glomerulonephritis, blood clots on the tiny filters of the glomerulus in the kidney. (Ancrod comes from the venom of vipers.)

Male hormones such as 19-nor testosterone and nandrolone—which do not have a masculinizing effect—may play a role in reducing disease activity. So far, the results of using such hormones have been mixed.

Immunoreplacement therapy is little more than a

concept at this point. This experimental approach involves "transplants," replacing very specific defective
immune components with healthy components.

Your Future with Lupus

No single volume can cover all the unique traits of
your disease. At best, the information in this book is a
starting point, or a turning point.

Make your new knowledge the basis for a better dia-
logue with your physician, who knows you best and who
should be a sounding board for any health decisions you
make.

Use your learning as a base to build on. There are
many excellent books on the subject; we've listed a few
in "Resources." Also, though fatigue may be a hallmark
symptom of lupus, the energy for support and education
seems almost limitless among people with lupus who
want to help. You'll find a support group in almost every
state. Linking up with national and local organizations—if only to receive their excellent and informative
newsletters—immediately connects you with a well-
spring of knowledge. See "Resources" for information.

At the very least, we hope *Living with Lupus* inspires
a more positive attitude about the disease, one that leads
toward a healthier and fuller life.

Resources

Organizations

American College of Rheumatology
60 Executive Park South, Suite 150
Atlanta, GA 30329
(404) 633-3777

American Lupus Society
3914 Del Amo Boulevard, Suite 922
Torrance, CA 90503
(310) 542-8891

Founded in 1973, ALS seeks to increase knowledge about lupus erythematosus. Through chapters and support groups, ALS aims to help lupus patients and their families cope with the daily problems associated with lupus. Local chapters hold meetings. ALS raises funds for research and actively works toward media awareness of lupus.

Publication: *Lupus Today*

Bay Area Lupus Foundation
Bay Area Chapter
2635 North First Street, Suite 206
San Jose, CA 95134
(408) 954-8600

Though a local chapter, BALF is an active organization
that sponsors many programs and publishes an excellent
newsletter. Though you may not be able to attend lectures, you may be able to get information the lectures
generate.

Publication: *newSLEtter*

Lupus Foundation of America
4 Research Plaza
Suite 180
Rockville, MD 20850-3226
(800) 558-0121

The mission of LFA is clear: to wipe out lupus. Toward
this goal, it funds research, conducts public awareness
programs, provides information and educational programs and lobbies lawmakers to fund appropriate research. Local support groups can be found across the
country; call headquarters for information.

Publication: *Lupus News*

Lupus Network
230 Ranch Drive
Bridgeport, CT 06606
(203) 372-5795

Founded in 1985, the Lupus Network is a coalition of
educators, medical professionals and individuals living
with lupus. It maintains a 200-volume library and distrib-
utes educational material, including an interesting news-

letter which combines personal observations and solutions with well-researched medical articles.

Publication: *Heliogram*

National Lupus Erythematosus Foundation
2635 North First Street, Suite 206
San Jose, CA 95134
(408) 954-8600

Founded in 1956, NLEF works to promote and encourage research into lupus. The group currently supports
research fellowships and clinics on lupus. In addition, it
maintains an advisory board of medical experts and tele-
phone counseling services.

National Institute of Arthritis and Musculoskeletal
and Skin Diseases (NIAMS) Centers

Part of the government's National Institutes of Health,
NIAMS seeks to develop and carry out programs in basic
and clinical research related to professional, patient and
public education. Though the scope of NIAMS extends
beyond lupus, NIAMS is the umbrella organization for
government-derived grants for lupus research. As a result, NIAMS is often on the cutting edge of new lupus
research. Difficult and complex cases are often referred
to these centers.

ALABAMA
University of Alabama at Birmingham
University Station
Birmingham, AL 34294
(205) 934-0542

CALIFORNIA
Division of Rheumatology
Ira Goldstein
W. M. Keck Autoimmune Disease Center

Department of Basic Clinical Research
Scripps Clinic & Research Foundation
10666 North Torrey Pines Road
La Jolla, CA 92037
(619) 457-8686

Stanford Arthritis Center
701 Welch Road, Suite 3301
Palo Alto, CA 94304
(415) 723-5907

CONNECTICUT
Division of Rheumatic Diseases
University of Connecticut School of Medicine
263 Farmington Avenue
Farmington, CT 06032
(203) 679-3290

MASSACHUSETTS
Boston University Arthritis Center
71 East Concord Street
Boston, MA 02118
(617) 414-5154

Brigham and Women's Hospital
75 Francis Street
Boston, MA 02115
(617) 732-5356

MICHIGAN
  Department of Internal Medicine
  1500 East Medical Center Drive
  Ann Arbor, MI 48109-0358
  (313) 936-4495

NEW YORK
  Multipurpose Arthritis Center
  Cornell Medical College
  S Building
  514 East 71st Street
  New York, NY 10021

NORTH CAROLINA
  Division of Rheumatology
  University of North Carolina School of Medicine
  932 Faculty Laboratory Office Building, Room 231H
  Chapel Hill, NC 27514
  (919) 966-4191

OHIO
  Division of Rheumatology
  Case Western Reserve University School of
    Medicine
  2073 Abington Road
  Cleveland, OH 44106
  (216) 844-3168

Pain Clinics

The following partial list includes clinics that specialize in managing chronic pain. Since they're devoted to pain in general, not lupus pain exclusively, these centers may not be able to help manage and treat the causes of pain in people with lupus. For centers closer to you, contact your local medical society.

CALIFORNIA
    City of Hope Medical Center
    Los Angeles, CA 90052

    Scripps Clinic
    Pain Treatment Center
    Claremont, CA 91711

    Cox Pain Center
    San Luis Obispo, CA 93401

    UCLA
    Pain Control Unit
    Los Angeles, CA 90024

    Division of Rheumatology
    University of California School of Medicine
    10833 Le Conte Avenue
    701 Welch Road, Suite 3301
    Palo Alto, CA 94304
    (415) 723-5907

FLORIDA
    Baptist Hospital
    Miami, FL 33101

Mount Sinai Hospital
Pain Consultation Center
Miami, FL 33101

University of Miami
School of Medicine
Pain Evaluation Team
Miami, FL 33101

GEORGIA
Emory University
Emory Clinic
Pain Control Center
Atlanta, GA 30333

ILLINOIS
University of Illinois
School of Medicine
Pain Clinic
Chicago, IL 60612

MARYLAND
Johns Hopkins School of Medicine
Pain Treatment Center
Baltimore, MD 21205

Mensana Clinic
Stevenson, MD 21153

NEW YORK
Pain Unit
Lourdes Hospital
Binghamton, NY 13902

NYU Medical Center
School of Medicine
New York, NY 10016

PENNSYLVANIA
University of Pittsburgh
Pain Control Center
Pittsburgh, PA 15261

TEXAS
Medical Center
Del Oro Hospital
Houston, TX 77002

VIRGINIA
University of Virginia Medical Center
Pain Clinic
Richmond, VA 23219

BOOKS

Look for these books at your public library, or contact
the Lupus Foundation of America for information. This is
by no means a complete list. Several excellent books—
including some directed at the medical community—are
available through LFA. Write to LFA at the address
given on page 181 for a complete catalog of publications.

Henrietta Aladjem, *Understanding Lupus*. New York:
Scribners, 1985. A thorough examination of medical
treatment and emotional issues, written with the aid of
more than twenty scientists and physicians.

Henrietta Aladjem and Peter Schur, M.D., *In Search of the Sun*. New York: Scribners, 1988. A double perspective on lupus from a patient and a physician.

Barbara Butler, *The Monster Under the Bed: Child Rearing When a Parent Is Chronically Ill*. Rockville, MD: Lupus Foundation of America, 1990. Examines the challenges to parenting with a chronic illness and offers commonsense solutions.

Margaret Erhart, *Augusta Cotton*. Cambridge, MA: Zoland, 1992. A novel dealing with the emotional trials and triumphs of a young girl with lupus.

Peggy Finton, *Parenting Plus: Raising Children with Special Health Needs*. New York: Dutton, 1990. Addresses the special challenges of raising children with chronic illness as well as other health problems.

Lupus Canada, *Lupus: The Disease with 1000 Faces*. Calgary, Alberta, Canada: Lupus Canada, 1990. A short, thorough guide to disease symptoms, emotional issues and treatments.

Peggy Maddox, *On the Edge: Health Crisis, Helping Yourself*. Lakewood, Colorado: Glenbridge, 1990.

Robert H. Phillips, Ph.D., *Coping with Lupus*. Garden City Park, NY: Avery Publishing Group, 1991. A compassionate guide through the emotional peaks and valleys of life with lupus.

Lydia Woods Schindler, *Understanding the Immune System*. Bethesda, MD: U.S. Department of Health and Human Services, 1988. Everything you wanted to know about the immune system, but could never understand before. Reading this pamphlet can be a challenge, but the struggle is worth it if you want to know about the immune system.

Jeannette M. Walters, *Introduction to Lupus and Disability Issues*. Rockville, MD: Lupus Foundation of America, 1990. A comprehensive guide to coping with Social Security, Medicare, Medicaid and other related issues.

Glossary

Acute—having a short course; not chronic

Adrenal glands—two small, triangular organs perched on top of the kidneys which make cortisol (corticosteroids) and other hormones

Albuminuria—protein in the urine

Allergen—any substance that causes allergy

Antibody—a protein made by B cells in response to the threat of a foreign substance; antibodies link up with antigen to form immune complexes

Antigen—a substance perceived by the immune system as being foreign and therefore potentially harmful

Antiinflammatory—any substance that acts to reduce inflammation, usually a medication

Antimalarial—a drug originally used for malaria that also eases symptoms of lupus, especially skin-related inflammation

Antinuclear antibodies (ANA)—antibodies that attack the nuclei of cells

Arthritis—an autoimmune reaction that causes inflammation of the joints

Aspirin—a pain- and inflammation-reducing drug

Autoantibody—antibody that attacks components of the body

Autoimmune—defending against the body's own parts

B cells—lymphocytes, or white cells, that come from bone marrow and produce antibodies; an essential part of the immune system

Biopsy—examination of a piece of body tissue under a microscope

Bone marrow—soft tissue at the center of bones that produces all blood cells

Butterfly rash—reddish lesions that cover the bridge of the nose and cheeks, in a shape resembling a butterfly (also called malar rash)

Chronic—lasting a long time

Complement—blood proteins important in the immune process that work along with antibodies by destroying bacteria, producing inflammation and helping to keep the immune system going

Corticosteroids—hormones made by the adrenal gland, as well as by drugs that mimic the natural hormone

Creatinine clearance test—a blood test that helps doctors monitor kidney health

Discoid lupus erythematosus—a form of lupus that mostly affects the skin and scalp

DNA (deoxyribonucleic acid)—a substance found in the nuclei of cells that transmits genetic information for that cell; it tells the cell what to be, what to do and how to do it

Drug-induced lupus—lupus reactions triggered by the use of certain drugs

Erythema and **erythematosus**—abnormal redness of the skin

Exacerbation—irritation; often means making worse, as in "exacerbation of symptoms"

False positive—a test result that reads as positive, but is really negative

Flare—a time when lupus symptoms appear or worsen, usually after a period without symptoms

Granulocytes—cell-eating white blood cells filled with granules that allow them to digest microorganisms; these cells help in the immune reaction by literally eating other organisms

Helper T cells—T cells that trigger the antibody reaction and stimulate immune response

Hematocrit (Hct)—a blood test used to measure the percentage of red blood cells in blood, usually expressed as a percentage of the total amount of blood

Hemoglobin (Hgb)—the protein in red blood cells that carries oxygen

Immune complex—a grouping of interlocking antibodies and antigen

Inflammation—swelling, redness and heat in response to infection

Late-onset lupus—lupus that occurs after a person's fiftieth year

LE cell—a cell found in the blood of up to 90 percent of people with lupus, but few people who do not have lupus

Local—confined to a specific area of the body; not system-wide

Lymphocytes—small white blood cells vital to the immune system

Neonatal lupus—a form of lupus that affects only newborns; most symptoms are mild and temporary (rash, nonthreatening changes in blood counts); in rare cases may cause life-threatening heart problems

Nonspecific—in disease, refers to symptoms that could be shared by many other conditions

NSAIDs—nonsteroidal antiinflammatory drugs, including aspirin and ibuprofen

Organism—a living thing

Photosensitivity—sensitivity to ultraviolet rays (from the sun and other light sources), which may cause skin or body-wide reactions

Plasma—the liquid portion of blood

Plasmapheresis—a procedure in which a machine filters out damaging cells and immune complexes from plasma

Pleurisy—inflammation of the lining of the lung

Prednisone, prednisolone—corticosteroid drugs

Proteinuria—excess of protein in the urine

Pulse steroid therapy—injection of high doses of corticosteroids for one or a few days in a row

Remission—a period during which a person is free of symptoms

Rheumatoid arthritis—a chronic immune system–related disease that causes inflammation of the joints

Serum—the clear liquid portion of blood, which serves as the home for antibodies (among other things)

Subacute cutaneous lupus erythematosus (SCLE) —a milder form of systemic and discoid lupus

Systemic—body-wide

Titer—the amount of a substance; usually refers to the amount of antibody

Urinalysis—analysis of the urine

Index

Page numbers in *italic* type indicate illustrations.